# Essentials of
# Medical Genetics for
# Health Professionals

**Laura M. Gunder, DHSc, MHE, PA-C**
Assistant Professor
Physician Assistant Department
School of Allied Health Sciences
Medical College of Georgia
Augusta, Georgia

Adjunct Faculty
Doctor of Health Sciences Program
Arizona School of Health Sciences
A.T. Still University
Mesa, Arizona

Staff Clinician
Peachtree Medical Center
Edgefield County Hospital
Ridge Spring, South Carolina

**Scott A. Martin, MS, PhD, PA-C**
Dean
Life Sciences Division
Athens Technical College
Athens, Georgia

Clinical Professor
Physician Assistant Department
School of Allied Health Sciences
Medical College of Georgia
Augusta, Georgia

Staff Clinician
Family Medicine
Athens, Georgia

D1511575

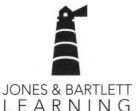

JONES & BARTLETT
LEARNING

*World Headquarters*

Jones & Bartlett Learning
40 Tall Pine Drive
Sudbury, MA 01776
978-443-5000
info@jblearning.com
www.jblearning.com

Jones & Bartlett Learning Canada
6339 Ormindale Way
Mississauga, Ontario L5V 1J2
Canada

Jones & Bartlett Learning International
Barb House, Barb Mews
London W6 7PA
United Kingdom

Jones & Bartlett Learning books and products are available through most bookstores and online booksellers. To contact Jones & Bartlett Learning directly, call 800-832-0034, fax 978-443-8000, or visit our website, www.jblearning.com.

Substantial discounts on bulk quantities of Jones & Bartlett Learning publications are available to corporations, professional associations, and other qualified organizations. For details and specific discount information, contact the special sales department at Jones & Bartlett Learning via the above contact information or send an email to specialsales@jblearning.com.

The authors, editor, and publisher have made every effort to provide accurate information. However, they are not responsible for errors, omissions, or for any outcomes related to the use of the contents of this book and take no responsibility for the use of the products and procedures described. Treatments and side effects described in this book may not be applicable to all people; likewise, some people may require a dose or experience a side effect that is not described herein. Drugs and medical devices are discussed that may have limited availability controlled by the Food and Drug Administration (FDA) for use only in a research study or clinical trial. Research, clinical practice, and government regulations often change the accepted standard in this field. When consideration is being given to use of any drug in the clinical setting, the health care provider or reader is responsible for determining FDA status of the drug, reading the package insert, and reviewing prescribing information for the most up-to-date recommendations on dose, precautions, and contraindications, and determining the appropriate usage for the product. This is especially important in the case of drugs that are new or seldom used.

**Production Credits**
Publisher: David Cella
Acquisitions Editor: Katey Birtcher
Associate Editor: Maro Gartside
Production Director: Amy Rose
Senior Production Editor: Renée Sekerak
Production Assistant: Sean Coombs
Marketing Manager: Grace Richards
Manufacturing and Inventory Control Supervisor: Amy Bacus
Assistant Photo Researcher: Rebecca Ritter
Composition: Auburn Associates, Inc.
Cover Design: Nancy Deutsch and Kristin E. Parker
Cover Images: Main image © Billy Lobo/ShutterStock, Inc.; Side images (from top to bottom) © Monkey Business Images/ Dreamstime.com; © Janpietruszka/Dreamstime.com; © Ron Chapple Studios/Dreamstime.com; © Monkey Business Images/ ShutterStock, Inc.
Printing and Binding: Malloy Incorporated
Cover Printing: Malloy Incorporated

**Library of Congress Cataloging-in-Publication Data**
Gunder, Laura M.
  Essentials of medical genetics for health professionals / Laura M. Gunder,
Scott A. Martin.
      p. ; cm.
  Includes bibliographical references and index.
  ISBN-13: 978-0-7637-5960-5 (pbk.)
  ISBN-10: 0-7637-5960-0 (pbk.)
  1. Medical genetics.  I. Martin, Scott A. II. Title.
  [DNLM: 1. Genetics, Medical. 2. Genetic Diseases, Inborn—diagnosis. 3.
Genetic Diseases, Inborn—therapy. QZ 50 G975e 2011]
  RB155.G895 2011
  616'.042—dc22
                              2010024290

6048
Printed in the United States of America
14  13  12      10 9 8 7 6 5 4 3

## DEDICATION

The profound privilege of being a healthcare provider revolves around our dedication to improving the human condition through our service to others. With the exception of our own families, we find our greatest joy in serving patients and their families as well as in mentoring and teaching students in our charge. This text is for the students, teachers, patients, colleagues, and families who seek to know more and serve better. May your knowledge and skills always be tempered by compassion, integrity, and humility—these virtues are essential to the character of a true servant.

## SPECIAL ACKNOWLEDGMENTS

Most often in one's career, it is the person's family that makes the greatest sacrifices. Families are unseen contributors in even our smallest accomplishments. This is certainly the case of those persons engaged in clinical practice, research, and academia, as working during many weekends, holidays, and evenings is required of us. Thank you all for your love, encouragement, and prayers and for making that sacrifice.

# Contents

# Preface

Learners enrolled in all healthcare training programs need to have a basic understanding of medical genetics so that they can successfully transition from students to clinicians. The field of medical genetics is advancing at a fast pace and is becoming increasingly integral to all aspects of medicine. This fact emphasizes the need for every practicing clinician and faculty member to develop an in-depth knowledge of the principles of human genetics, given that they are applicable to such a wide variety of clinical presentations. Underscoring that importance, effective September 2006, the Accreditation Review Commission on Education for Physician Assistants (ARC-PA) requires that medical genetics be included in the curriculum of every PA program.

Likewise, there is a need to train primary care providers and related health professionals to meet the growing demand for genetic intervention. Although genetic counselors typically address most questions asked by the patient and family when a genetic test result is received, it falls to the primary care clinician and those involved in the direct patient care to address the same issues recurrently over the patient's lifetime. With the Human Genome Project progressing rapidly, and sequencing of the human genome being completed ahead of schedule, genetic conditions and their multifactorial nature are increasingly requiring that treatment and prevention measures become highly individualized. The primary care provider in particular stands at the frontline of this interface and will play an integral role in intervention and prevention of genetically based diseases.

The incorporation of medical genetics into medical education and residency training programs has also begun. However, because the understanding of genomics is relatively new, a gap exists between the education and training of those practicing clinicians, the existing curriculum, and the integration of the principles into clinical practice. Curriculum guidelines exist to assist developers and educators in integrating medical genetics into the existing curricula for most disciplines.

Because the concepts and principles of medical genetics are multidisciplinary and complex, it is especially important to consider the most efficient and effective methods of delivery of genetics-related education during the program planning. In addition to genetic diseases and disorders, the program should include an appreciation of the rapid advances in genetics, the need for lifelong learning, the need for referral, and the role of genetic counselors and medical geneticists. On a practical level, it should ensure that students develop the ability to construct and analyze a three-generation pedigree.

This text is intended to serve as the basis for a medical genetics curriculum that provides an opportunity for students to integrate genetic knowledge, skills, and attitudes early in their medical education and training. Other benefits of the text include improved student understanding of genetic concepts in clinical medicine and improved clinical skills, which will ultimately translate into improved patient outcomes. It is further recommended that PA faculty and other medical educators receive formal instruction in medical genetics education.

This text is designed to introduce the discipline of clinical genetics to physician assistant students, medical students, and other healthcare providers. While many other genetics texts are available, most are inappropriate for the accelerated curriculum associated with PA programs. Students have commented that many of these texts are very cumbersome and too detailed, requiring too much time to extract the most important clinical information. Accordingly, the overarching goal of this book is to assist the reader in making the transition from knowledge-based learning in the didactic curriculum to competency-based practice in the clinical training period and beyond. Moreover, it aims to encourage all practicing providers to integrate their new knowledge, skills, and attitudes related to the latest medical genetics into their everyday clinical practice.

To achieve these ends, the approach taken toward the specific disorders profiled in this text includes an explanation of the genetics involved, signs and symptoms of the disease, treatment and management options, and disease surveillance. A brief review of chromosomes, DNA, RNA, protein synthesis, inheritance patterns, diagnostic techniques, embryonic development, and teratogens is also provided. Finally, the roles of genetic counseling and screening, and an introduction to some ethical and legal issues related to medical genetics, are included. Keeping in mind that many faculty will seek out this text as the foundation for a course in clinically relevant medical genetics, this book covers selected topics encountered in a primary care setting that may be ameliorated by early diagnosis and intervention and that cover every organ system.

This book is written in a simple-to-read format that avoids excessive use of genetics jargon. Chapters cover disease topics in all organ systems, ensuring that the text can be used in a variety of curricular formats—either as the sole text in a stand-alone course or as a supplemental resource for teaching clinical medicine in an organ system format across the curriculum. *Please realize that this book is not meant to be an all-inclusive textbook on genetics, as many such books are readily available today.* You will find that this text not only has application in the classroom setting for allied health students and medical students, but is also clinically useful and timely for practicing clinicians (i.e., physician assistants, nurse practitioners, physicians, nurses) who want to learn more and stay abreast of new information in the area of genetics.

Many of the chapters offer a list of resources including many Web site addresses, given that most students and providers today are likely to access a peer-reviewed Web site to obtain the most up-to-date medical information. Tables, figures, chapter summaries, and chapter review questions assist the reader in extracting the most pertinent information in a timely manner.

We hope that students and clinicians will find this text to be a concise, user-friendly, and clinically relevant read.

*L. M. Gunder*

# Chapter 1

# Introduction

## CHAPTER OBJECTIVES

✓ Review molecular genetics and associated terminology.
✓ Review Mendelian genetic principles.
✓ Define mutation and give examples of different types of mutations.
✓ Describe different inheritance patterns.

The goal of this chapter is not to go into exhaustive genetic detail, but to familiarize the reader with basic genetic concepts (e.g., meiosis and mitosis, haploid versus diploid) by providing a basic overview of molecular genetics, simple inheritance patterns, chromosomal aberrations, and mutations. For more detailed information or to refresh your memory, the reader is referred to any one of a number of comprehensive genetics textbooks. The following texts are all recommended:

- Hartl DL, Jones EW. *Genetics: Analysis of Genes and Genomes,* 6th ed. Sudbury, MA: Jones and Bartlett; 2005.
- Jameson JL, Kopp P. Principles of Human Genetics. In: Fauci AS, Braunwald E, Kasper DL, Hauser SL, Longo DL, Jameson JL, Loscalzo J (Eds.), Harrison's *Principles of Internal Medicine,* 17th ed. New York: McGraw-Hill Medical; 2008.
- Jorde LB, Carey JC, Bamshad MJ, White RL. *Medical Genetics,* 3rd ed. St. Louis, MO: Mosby; 2006.
- Mange EJ, Mange AP. *Basic Human Genetics.* Sunderland, MA: Sinauer Associates; 1994.
- Singer M, Berg P. *Genes and Genomes: A Changing Perspective.* Mill Valley, CA: University Science Books; 1991.

## Basic Genetics

Genetics is the study of biologically inherited traits determined by elements of heredity that are transmitted from parents to offspring in reproduction. These inherited elements are called **genes**. Recent advances in the field of **genomics** have led to development of methods that can determine the complete **deoxyribonucleic acid (DNA)** sequence of an organism. Genomics is the latest advance in the study of the chemical nature of genes and the ways that genes function to affect certain traits.

The work of Gregor Mendel, a monk and part-time biologist, with garden peas is regarded as the beginning of what would become the science of genetics. Mendel is credited with showing the existence of genes as well as illuminating the rules governing their transmission from generation to generation. The study of genetics through the analysis of offspring from matings is sometimes referred to as classical genetics.

The billions of nucleotides in the nucleus of a cell are organized linearly along the DNA double helix in functional units called genes. Each of the 20,000 to 25,000 human genes is accompanied by various regulatory elements that control when that gene is active in producing **messenger ribonucleic acid (mRNA)** by the process of **transcription**. In most situations, mRNA is transported from the nucleus to the cytoplasm, where its genetic information is used in the manufacture of proteins (a process called **translation**), which perform the functions that ultimately determine phenotype. For example, proteins serve as enzymes that facilitate metabolism and cell synthesis; as DNA binding elements that regulate transcription of other genes; as structural elements of cells and the extracellular matrix; and as receptor molecules for intracellular and intercellular communication. DNA also encodes many small RNA molecules that serve functions that are not yet fully understood, including regulating gene transcription and interfering with the translational capacity of some mRNAs.

**Chromosomes** are the means by which the genes are transmitted from generation to generation. Each chromosome is a complex of protein and nucleic acid in which an unbroken double helix of DNA is tightly wound (**Figure 1-1**). Genes are found along the length of chromosomes. A variety of highly complicated and integrated processes occur within

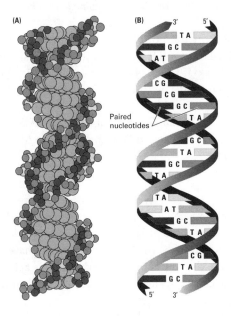

**Figure 1-1** Molecular structure of a DNA double helix. (A) A space-filling model in which each atom is depicted as a sphere. (B) A diagram highlighting the helical backbones on the outside of the molecule and stacked A-T and G-C pairs inside.

the chromosome, including DNA replication, recombination, and transcription. In the nucleus of each of their somatic cells, humans normally have 46 chromosomes, which are arranged in 23 pairs. One of these pairs, consisting of the **sex chromosomes** X and Y, determines the sex of the individual; females have the pair XX and males have the pair XY. The remaining 22 pairs of chromosomes are called **autosomes**. In addition to these nuclear chromosomes, each mitochondrion (an organelle found in varying numbers in the cytoplasm of all cells) contains multiple copies of a small chromosome. This **mitochondrial chromosome** encodes a few of the proteins for oxidative metabolism and all of the **transfer ribonucleic acids (tRNA)** used in translation of proteins within this organelle. Mitochondrial chromosomes are inherited almost entirely from the cytoplasm of the fertilized ovum and, therefore, are maternal in origin.

The exact location of a gene on a chromosome is known as its **locus**, and the array of loci constitutes the human gene map. Currently, researchers have identified the chromosomal sites of more than 11,000 genes (i.e., those for which normal or abnormal function has been identified).

Homologous copies of a gene are termed **alleles**. In comparing alleles, it must be specified at which level of analysis the comparison is being made. For example, if alleles are truly identical, their coding sequences and the number of copies do not vary, so the individual is **homozygous** at that specific locus. However, if the DNA is analyzed using either restriction enzyme examination or nucleotide sequencing, then, despite having the same functional identity, the alleles would be viewed as different and the individual would be **heterozygous** for that locus. Heterozygosity based on differences in the protein products of alleles has been detectable for decades and represents the first hard evidence proving the high degree of human biologic variability. In the past decade, analysis of DNA sequences has shown genetic variability to be much more common, with differences in nucleotide sequence between individuals occurring about once every 1200 nucleotides.

## Mutation

A **mutation** is defined as a change in DNA that may adversely affect the host. A heterozygous allele frequently results when different alleles are inherited from the egg and the sperm, but it may also occur as a consequence of spontaneous alteration in nucleotide sequence that results in a mutation. A **germinal mutation** occurs during formation of an egg or a sperm. If the change occurs after conception, it is termed a **somatic mutation**. The role of somatic mutation is now increasingly recognized as a key factor in the etiology of human disease.

The most dramatic type of mutation is an alteration in the number or physical structure of chromosomes, a phenomenon called a **chromosomal aberration**. Not all aberrations cause problems in the affected individual, but some that do not may lead to problems in their offspring. Approximately 1 in every 200 live-born infants has a chromosomal aberration that is detected because of some effect on phenotype. The frequency of this finding increases markedly the earlier in fetal life that the chromosomes are examined. By the end of the first trimester of gestation, most fetuses with abnormal numbers of chromosomes have been lost through spontaneous abortion.

For example, during the reduction division of meiosis that leads to production of mature ova and sperm, failure of chromosome pairs to separate in the dividing cell (**nondisjunction**) causes the embryo to have too many or too few chromosomes. When this type of error occurs, it is called **aneuploidy**, and either more or fewer than 46 chromosomes are present. Three types of aneuploidy may occur: (1) **monosomy**, in which only one member of a pair of chromosomes is present; (2) **trisomy**, in which three chromosomes are present instead of two; and (3) **polysomy**, in which one chromosome is represented four or more times.

During **translocation** or **inversion**, there is a rearrangement of chromosome arms. This effect is considered a mutation even if breakage and reunion do not disrupt any coding sequence (**Figures 1-2 and 1-3**). In an inversion, a chromosomal region becomes

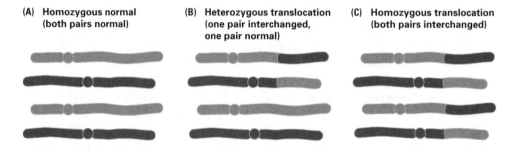

**(A) Homozygous normal (both pairs normal)**

**(B) Heterozygous translocation (one pair interchanged, one pair normal)**

**(C) Homozygous translocation (both pairs interchanged)**

**Figure 1-2** (A) Two pairs of nonhomologous chromosomes in a diploid organism. (B) Heterozygous reciprocal translocation in which two nonhomologous chromosomes (the two at the top) have interchanged terminal segments. (C) Homozygous reciprocal translocation.

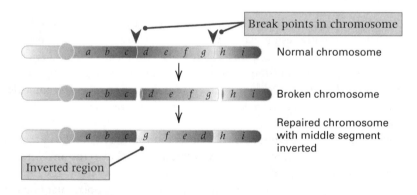

**Figure 1-3** Origin of an inversion by reversal of the region between two chromosomal break points.

reoriented 180 degrees out of the ordinary phase. In each case, the same genetic material is present, but appears in a different order. Consequently, the phenotypic effect of gross chromosomal mutations can range from profound (as in aneuploidy) to innocuous.

Less obvious, but still detectable cytologically, are **deletions** of part of a chromosome. These mutations almost always alter phenotype, because a number of genes are lost. However, a deletion may involve only a single nucleotide, whereas 1 to 2 million nucleotides (1 to 2 megabases) must be lost before the defect can be visualized by the most sensitive cytogenetic methods. More sensitive molecular biology techniques are needed to detect smaller losses.

Changes in one nucleotide can alter which amino acid is encoded. For example, if the amino acid is present in a critical region of the protein, normal protein function might be severely disrupted (e.g., sickle cell disease; see Chapter 9). In contrast, some other amino acid substitutions have no detectable effect on function, such that the phenotype is unaltered by the mutation. Also, within the genetic code, two or more different three-nucleotide sequences called **codons** may encode the same amino acids (**degenerate**), such that nucleotide substitution does not necessarily alter the amino acid sequence of the protein. Three specific codons signal termination of translation, so a nucleotide substitution that generates one of the stop codons prematurely usually causes a **truncated protein**, which is frequently abnormal.

## Nondisjunction Syndromes

Mutations may occur spontaneously or may be induced by radiation, medication, viral infections, or other environmental factors. Both advanced maternal and paternal age are associated with different types of mutations. In women, meiosis is completed only when an egg ovulates, and chromosomal nondisjunction is increasingly common as the egg becomes older. An example is trisomy 21, also known as **Down syndrome**. The risk that an aneuploid egg will result increases exponentially and becomes a major clinical concern for women older than their early 30s who wish to conceive a child (**Figure 1-4**). In men, mutations affecting nucleotide sequences are more subtle and increase with age. Offspring of men older than 40 years of age are at an increased risk for having primarily **autosomal dominant** Mendelian conditions.

Down syndrome is one of the most common trisomies, with approximately 1 of every 800 babies born in the United States being affected by this condition, which includes a combination of birth defects. Affected individuals have some degree of mental retardation, characteristic facial features, and, often, heart defects and other health problems. They are typically short with round, moonlike faces (**Figure 1-5**). Their tongues protrude forward, forcing their mouths open, and their eyes slant upward at the corners. The severity of these problems varies greatly among affected individuals.

Some of the health problems associated with Down syndrome are shown in **Table 1-1**. Fortunately, most are treatable. Thus life expectancy for persons with trisomy 21 is now approximately 55 years. The degree of mental retardation varies from mild to severe.

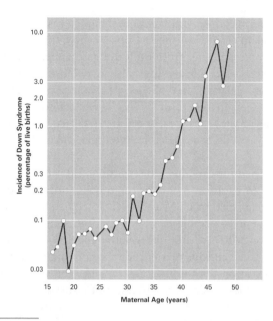

**Figure 1-4** Frequency of Down syndrome (number of cases per 100 live births) related to age of mother. The graph is based on 438 Down syndrome births (among 330,859 total births) in Sweden in the period 1968 to 1970.

*Source:* Data from Hook EB, Lindsjö A. *American Journal of Human Genetics.* 30:19; 1978.

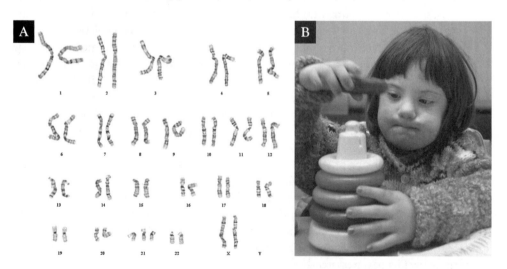

**Figure 1-5** Down syndrome. (A) Karyotype of Down syndrome girl with trisomy of chromosome 21. (B) Distinguishing characteristics of Down syndrome.

*Source:* (A) Courtesy of Viola Freeman, Associate Professor, Faculty of Health Sciences, Dept. of Pathology and Molecular Medicine, McMaster University. (B) © PhotoCreate/ShutterStock, Inc.

Table 1-1    **Health Problems Associated with Down Syndrome**

| Problem | Specifics | Recommendation |
|---|---|---|
| Heart defects | Almost half of babies have heart defects. | Babies should be examined by a pediatric cardiologist and have an echocardiogram in the first 2 months of life. |
| Intestinal defects | Approximately 12% of babies are born with intestinal malformations that require surgery. | |
| Vision problems | Crossed eyes, near- or far-sightedness, and cataracts. | Babies should have a pediatric ophthalmologist exam within the first 6 months of life and have regular vision exams. |
| Hearing loss | Approximately 75% of children have some hearing loss. It may be due to fluid in the middle ear (which may be temporary), a nerve, or both. | Babies should be screened for hearing loss at birth or by 3 months of age as well as have regular exams. |
| Infections | Children tend to have many colds and ear infections as well as bronchitis and pneumonia. | Children should receive all the standard childhood immunizations. |
| Memory loss | Affected individuals more likely than unaffected individuals to develop Alzheimer's disease at an earlier age. | |

*Source:* Adapted from Down syndrome. Pregnancy & Newborn Health Education Center. March of Dimes Web site. http://www.marchofdimes.com/pnhec/4439_1214.asp. Accessed January 16, 2010.

Because severe mental retardation is less likely, many affected individuals are able to go to school and participate in special work programs.

The American College of Obstetricians and Gynecologists recommends that all pregnant women be offered a screening test for Down syndrome, regardless of the woman's age. Screening may consist of a maternal blood test done in the first trimester (at 11 to 13 weeks of pregnancy), along with a special ultrasound examination of the back of the baby's neck (called nuchal translucency), or a maternal blood test done in the second trimester (at 15 to 20 weeks of pregnancy). These tests help to identify pregnancies that are at higher-than-average risk of Down syndrome, but cannot diagnose Down syndrome or other birth defects.

Women who have an abnormal screening test result are offered a diagnostic test, such as **amniocentesis** or **chorionic villus sampling** (CVS), that will either confirm or disprove the presence of Down syndrome in the fetus. Amniocentesis involves the removal and examination of a small sample of the amniotic fluid that surrounds the fetus. Chorionic villus sampling involves taking a tiny tissue sample from outside the sac where the fetus develops (chorionic villi) and is done earlier in pregnancy (usually between 10 and 12 weeks) than amniocentesis (usually 15 to 20 weeks). Both procedures pose a small risk of miscarriage, with CVS having a slightly higher risk than amniocentesis. These tests are highly accurate at diagnosing or ruling out Down syndrome.

Nondisjunction of the sex chromosomes can lead to a variety of nonlethal genetic disorders. One of the most common occurs when an ovum with an extra X chromosome is fertilized by a sperm with a Y chromosome. This process results in an XXY genotype, known as **Klinefelter syndrome**. Klinefelter syndrome occurs in approximately 1 out of every 700 to 1000 newborn males. Even though these individuals are males, their masculinization is incomplete. Their external genitalia and testes are unusually small, and approximately 50% of these individuals develop breasts. Spermatogenesis is abnormal, and affected males are generally sterile. Klinefelter syndrome is the most common chromosomal disorder associated with male hypogonadism and infertility.

Another disorder associated with nondisjunction of sex chromosomes is **Turner syndrome**. This monosomy syndrome results when an ovum lacking the X chromosome is fertilized by a sperm that contains an X chromosome. It may also occur when a genetically normal ovum is fertilized by a sperm lacking an X or Y chromosome. The result is an offspring with 22 pairs of autosomes and a single, unmatched X chromosome (XO).

Turner syndrome occurs in only 1 out of every 10,000 female births, as the XO embryo is more likely to be spontaneously aborted. These individuals look like females and are characteristically short with wide chests and a prominent fold of skin on their necks. Because their ovaries fail to develop at puberty, they are sterile and have low levels of estrogen and small breasts. Mental retardation is not associated with this disorder, so individuals lead fairly normal lives.

## Genes in Individuals

Most human characteristics and common diseases are **polygenic**, whereas many of the disordered phenotypes thought of as "genetic" are **monogenic** but still influenced by other loci in a person's genome. Phenotypes due to alterations at a single gene are frequently referred to as **Mendelian**, after Gregor Mendel, the monk/biologist who studied the reproducibility and recurrence of variation in garden peas. Mendel showed that some traits were **dominant** relative to other traits; he called the latter traits **recessive**. Dominant traits require only one copy of a "factor" to be expressed, regardless of what the other copy is, whereas recessive traits require two copies before expression occurs. We now recognize that the Mendelian factors are genes, and the alternative copies of the gene are alleles. For example, if $B$ is the common (normal) allele and $b$ is the mutant allele at a locus, then the phenotype is dominant whether the genotype is $BB$ or $Bb$. Conversely, the phenotype is recessive when the genotype is $bb$.

# Inheritance Patterns

As described earlier, phenotypes due to alterations at a single gene are characterized as Mendelian and monogenic human diseases are frequently referred to as Mendelian disorders. The mode of inheritance for a given phenotypic trait or disease is determined by **pedigree analysis**. All affected and unaffected individuals in the family are recorded in a pedigree using standard symbols (**Figure 1-6**). The principles of allelic segregation, and the transmission of alleles from parents to children, are illustrated in **Figure 1-7**. One

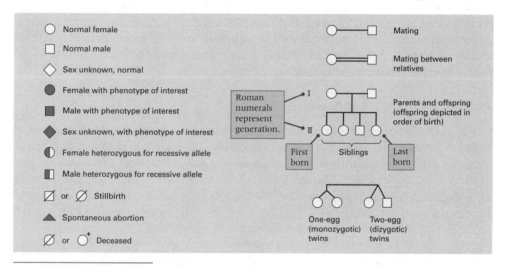

**Figure 1-6** Conventional symbols used in depicting human pedigrees.
*Source:* Bennett R, French K, Resta R, Doyle D. Standardized Human Pedigree Nomenclature: Update and Assessment of the Recommendations of the National Society of Genetic Counselors. *Journal of Genetic Counseling.* 17:424–433;2008. ©National Society of Genetic Counselors, Inc. 2008.

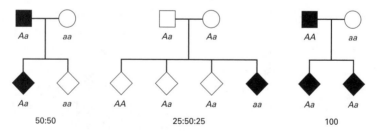

**Figure 1-7** Segregation of genotypes in the offspring of parents with one dominant (A) and one recessive (*a*) allele. The distribution of the parental alleles to their offspring depends on the combination present in the parents. Filled symbols = affected individuals.
*Source:* Reproduced from Fauci AS, Kasper DL, Braunwald E, Hauser SI, Longo DL, Jameson JL, Loscalzo J. *Harrison's Principles of Internal Medicine*, 17th ed; 2008. http:www.accessmedicine.com. Copyright © The McGraw-Hill Companies, Inc. All rights reserved.

dominant (*A*) allele and one recessive (*a*) allele can display any of three Mendelian modes of inheritance: autosomal dominant, autosomal recessive, or chromosome X-linked. Approximately 65% of human monogenic disorders are autosomal dominant, 25% are autosomal recessive, and 5% are X-linked. Genetic testing is now available for many of these disorders and plays an increasingly important role in clinical medicine.

## Autosomal Dominant Inheritance

Autosomal dominant disorders are relevant because mutations in a single allele are sufficient to cause the disease (**Figure 1-8**). In contrast to recessive disorders, in which disease pathogenesis is relatively straightforward because there is loss of gene function, dominant disorders can be caused by various disease mechanisms, many of which are unique to the function of the genetic pathway involved.

## Autosomal Recessive Inheritance

In the case of recessive disorders, mutated alleles result in a complete or partial loss of function. An example pedigree of autosomal recessive inheritance is shown in **Figure 1-9**. Recessive disorders frequently involve enzymes in metabolic pathways, receptors, or proteins in signaling cascades. The affected individual can be of either sex and either a homozygote or compound heterozygote for a single-gene defect. Fortunately, autosomal recessive diseases are, for the most part, rare and often occur in the context of parental

### CHARACTERISTICS OF AUTOSOMAL DOMINANT INHERITANCE

- A vertical pattern is observed in the pedigree, with multiple generations being affected.
- Heterozygotes for the mutant allele show an abnormal phenotype.
- Males and females are affected with equal frequency and severity.
- Only one parent must be affected for an offspring to be at risk for developing the phenotype.
- When an affected person mates with an unaffected one, each offspring has a 50% chance of inheriting the affected phenotype. This is true regardless of the sex of the affected parent—specifically, male-to-male transmission occurs.
- The frequency of sporadic cases is positively associated with the severity of the phenotype. Autosomal dominant phenotypes are often age dependent, less severe than autosomal recessive phenotypes, and associated with malformations or other physical features.

*Source:* Reproduced from Pyeritz RE. Medical Genetics. In Tierney L, et al. *Current Medical Diagnosis & Treatment*, 42nd ed. 2003.

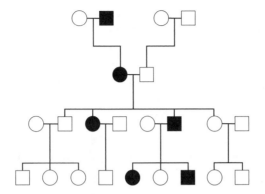

**Figure 1-8** A pedigree illustrating autosomal dominant inheritance. Square symbols indicate males and circles indicate females; open symbols indicate that the person is phenotypically unaffected, and filled symbols indicate that the phenotype is present to some extent.
*Source:* Reproduced from Tierney L, et al. *Current Medical Diagnosis & Treatment*, 42nd ed; 2003. Copyright © The McGraw-Hill Companies, Inc. All rights reserved.

**consanguinity**. The relatively high frequency of certain recessive disorders, such as sickle cell anemia (see Chapter 9), cystic fibrosis (see Chapter 11), and thalassemia (see Chapter 9), is partially explained by a selective biologic advantage for the heterozygous state. Heterozygous carriers of a defective allele are usually clinically normal, but they may display subtle differences in phenotype that become apparent only with more precise testing or in the context of certain environmental influences (i.e., sickle cell disease; see Chapter 9).

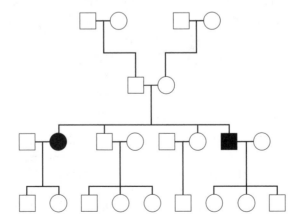

**Figure 1-9** A pedigree illustrating autosomal recessive inheritance.
*Source:* Reproduced from Tierney L, et al. *Current Medical Diagnosis & Treatment*, 42nd ed; 2003. Copyright © The McGraw-Hill Companies, Inc. All rights reserved.

Autosomal recessive phenotypes are often associated with deficient activity of enzymes and are thus termed **inborn errors of metabolism**. Such disorders include phenylketonuria, Tay-Sachs disease, and the various glycogen storage diseases. They tend to be more severe, less variable, and less age dependent than dominant conditions. When an autosomal recessive condition is quite rare, the chance that the parents of affected offspring are consanguineous for the phenotype is increased. As a result, the prevalence of rare recessive conditions is high among inbred groups such as the Old Order Amish and Ashkenazi Jews.

## CHARACTERISTICS OF AUTOSOMAL RECESSIVE INHERITANCE

- A horizontal pattern is noted in the pedigree, with a single generation being affected.

- Males and females are affected with equal frequency and severity.

- Inheritance is from both parents, each of whom is a heterozygote (carrier) and each of whom is usually clinically unaffected by his or her carrier status.

- Each offspring of two carriers has a 25% chance of being affected, a 50% chance of being a carrier, and a 25% chance of inheriting neither mutant allele. Thus two-thirds of all clinically unaffected offspring are carriers of the autosomal recessive phenotype.

- In matings between individuals, each with the same recessive phenotype, all offspring will be affected.

- Affected individuals who mate with unaffected individuals who are not carriers have only unaffected offspring.

- The rarer the recessive phenotype, the more likely it is that the parents are consanguineous (related).

*Source:* Reproduced from Pyeritz RE. Medical Genetics. In Tierney L, et al. *Current Medical Diagnosis & Treatment*, 42nd ed. 2003.

## X-Linked Inheritance

Because males have only one X chromosome, a daughter will always inherit her father's X chromosome in addition to one of her mother's two X chromosomes (**Figure 1-10**). Conversely, a son inherits the Y chromosome from his father and one maternal X chromosome, so the risk of developing disease due to a mutant X-chromosomal gene differs in the two sexes. Due to the presence of one X chromosome, males are said to be **hemizygous** for the mutant allele on that chromosome. Therefore, they are more likely to develop the mutant phenotype, regardless of whether the mutation is dominant or recessive. A female with two X chromosomes may be either heterozygous or homozygous for the mutant allele, which may be dominant or recessive. Therefore, the terms "X-linked dominant" and "X-linked recessive" are applicable to expression of the mutant phenotype only in women.

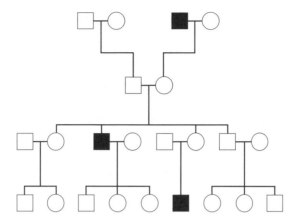

**Figure 1-10**  A pedigree illustrating X-linked inheritance.

*Source:* Reproduced from Tierney L, et al. *Current Medical Diagnosis & Treatment*, 42nd ed; 2003. Copyright © The McGraw-Hill Companies, Inc. All rights reserved.

## CHARACTERISTICS OF X-LINKED INHERITANCE

- There is no male-to-male transmission of the phenotype.
- Unaffected males do not transmit the phenotype.
- All daughters of an affected male are heterozygous carriers.
- Males are usually more severely affected than females.
- Whether a heterozygous female is counted as affected—and whether the phenotype is called "recessive" or "dominant"—often depends on the sensitivity of the assay or examination.
- Some mothers of affected males will not themselves be heterozygotes (i.e., they will be homozygous normal) but will have a germinal mutation. The proportion of heterozygous (carrier) mothers is negatively associated with the severity of the condition.
- Heterozygous women transmit the mutant gene to 50% of their sons, who are affected, and to 50% of their daughters, who are heterozygotes.
- If an affected male mates with a heterozygous female, 50% of the male offspring will be affected, giving the false impression of male-to-male transmission. Among the female offspring of such matings, 50% will be affected as severely as the average hemizygous male; in small pedigrees, this pattern may simulate autosomal dominant inheritance.

*Source:* Reproduced from Pyeritz RE. Medical Genetics. In Tierney L, et al. *Current Medical Diagnosis & Treatment*, 42nd ed. 2003.

The characteristics of X-linked inheritance depend on phenotypic severity. For some disorders, affected males do not survive to reproduce. In such cases, approximately two-thirds of affected males have a carrier mother; in the remaining third, the disorder arises by new germinal mutation in an X chromosome of the mother. When the disorder is nearly always manifested in heterozygous females (X-linked dominant inheritance), females tend to be affected approximately twice as often as males; on average, an affected female transmits the phenotype to 50% of her sons and 50% of her daughters.

The Y chromosome has a relatively small number of genes. One gene, the sex-region determining Y factor (*SRY*), encodes the testis-determining factor that is crucial for normal male development. Normally there is infrequent exchange of sequences on the Y chromosome with the X chromosome.

## Mitochondrial Inheritance

As described earlier, transmission of genes encoded by DNA contained in the nuclear chromosomes follows the principles of Mendelian inheritance. In addition, each mitochondrion contains several copies of a small circular chromosome that encodes tRNA, **ribosomal RNA (rRNA)**, and proteins that are involved in oxidative phosphorylation and ATP generation. The mitochondrial genome does not recombine and is inherited through the maternal line because sperm does not contribute significant cytoplasmic

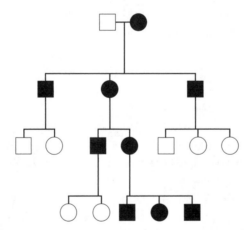

**Figure 1-11** Mitochondrial ("maternal") inheritance. A mitochondrial genetic mutation, indicated by darkened symbols, is passed by the female (circle) to all of her offspring, including males (squares). Among the subsequent offspring, the males do not transmit the mutation, but the females continue to transmit the mutation to all of their offspring because mitochondria are passed through ova, not sperm.
*Source:* Reproduced from Pyeritz RE. Chapter e2: Basic Genetics. McPhee SJ, Papadakis MA, Tierney LM, Jr. *Current Medical Diagnosis & Treatment,* 48th ed; 2009. http:www.accessmedicine.com/content. aspx?aID=774551. Copyright © The McGraw-Hill Companies, Inc. All rights reserved.

components to the zygote. Mutations in the genes encoded by the mitochondrial chromosome cause a variety of diseases that affect (in particular) organs highly dependent on oxidative metabolism, such as the retina, brain, kidneys, and heart. An affected woman can pass the defective mitochondrial chromosome to all of her offspring, whereas an affected man has little risk of passing his mutation to a child (**Figure 1-11**).

## Human Genome Project

Genomics is the study of all the genes in a person as well as the interactions of these genes with one another and with the individual's environment. All people are 99.9% identical in genetic makeup, but differences in the remaining 0.1% offer important clues about health and disease. The goals of the Human Genome Project were to determine the complete sequence of the 3 billion DNA subunits (bases), identify all human genes, and make that information accessible for further biological study. The project was completed in 2003 and identified approximately 25,000 genes in human DNA.

### GENOMIC SEQUENCING HIGHLIGHTS

- The human genome contains 3.2 billion chemical nucleotide bases (A, C, T, and G).
- The average gene consists of 3000 bases, but sizes vary greatly. The largest known human gene is dystrophin, which has 2.4 million base pairs.
- Functions are unknown for more than 50% of discovered genes.
- The human genome sequence is almost exactly (99.9%) the same in all people.
- Approximately 2% of the genome encodes instructions for the synthesis of proteins.
- Repeat sequences that do not code for proteins make up at least 50% of the human genome.
- Repeat sequences are thought to have no direct functions, but they shed light on chromosome structure and dynamics. Over time, these repeats reshape the genome by rearranging it, thereby creating entirely new genes or modifying and reshuffling existing genes.
- The human genome has a much greater portion (50%) of repeat sequences than the mustard weed (11%), the worm (7%), and the fly (3%).
- More than 40% of the predicted human proteins share similarity with fruit-fly or worm proteins.
- Genes appear to be concentrated in random areas along the genome, with vast expanses of noncoding DNA occurring between these areas.

*Continued*

- Chromosome 1 (the largest human chromosome) has the most genes (3168), and the Y chromosome has the fewest (344).
- Particular gene sequences have been associated with numerous diseases and disorders, including breast cancer, muscle disease, deafness, and blindness.
- Scientists have identified millions of locations where single-base DNA differences occur in humans. This information promises to revolutionize the processes of finding DNA sequences associated with such common diseases as cardiovascular disease, diabetes, arthritis, and cancers.

*Source:* U.S. Department of Energy Genome Programs, Insights from the Human DNA Sequence. Available at http://www.ornl.gov/sci/techresources/Human_Genome/publicat/primer2001/4.shtml. Accessed August 13, 2010.

The completion of the Human Genome Project has inspired much excitement regarding the many potential applications using this information: (1) improved disease diagnosis, (2) ability to detect genetic predispositions to disease, (3) development of drugs based on molecular information, (4) use of gene therapy and control systems as drugs, and (5) creation of "custom drugs" based on individual genetic profiles. In addition, the creation of more detailed genome maps has helped researchers seeking genes associated with dozens of genetic conditions, including myotonic dystrophy, fragile X syndrome, neurofibromatosis types 1 and 2, inherited colon cancer, Alzheimer's disease, and familial breast cancer. Even though the concept of using this genetic information to treat and/or cure many diseases is very exciting, many challenges must be overcome before viable and safe treatments are available for human diseases.

## Chapter Summary

- Genetics is the study of biologically inherited traits determined by genes that are transmitted from parents to offspring during the course of reproduction.
- Chromosomes are how the genes are transmitted from generation to generation.
- The human genome is estimated to contain 20,000 to 25,000 genes. A germinal mutation occurs during formation of an egg or a sperm, but if change occurs after conception it is termed a somatic mutation.
- Advanced maternal and paternal age are associated with different types of mutations.
- Phenotypes due to alterations at a single gene are characterized as Mendelian, and monogenic human diseases are frequently referred to as Mendelian disorders.
- Genomics is the study of all the genes in a person as well as the interactions of these genes with one another and with an individual's environment.

## Key Terms

**Allele:** any of the alternative forms of a given gene.

**Amniocentesis:** a prenatal test in which a small sample of the amniotic fluid surrounding the fetus is removed and examined.

**Aneuploidy:** a condition in which extra or fewer copies of particular genes or chromosomal regions are present compared with the wild type.

**Autosomal dominant:** a pattern of inheritance in which an affected individual has one copy of a mutant gene and one normal gene on a pair of autosomal chromosomes. Individuals with autosomal dominant diseases have a 50:50 chance of passing the mutant gene—and, therefore, the disorder—on to each of their children.

**Autosomes:** all chromosomes other than the sex chromosomes.

**Chorionic villus sampling (CVS):** a prenatal test that involves taking a tiny tissue sample from outside the sac where the fetus develops. It is performed between 10 and 12 weeks after a now-pregnant woman's last menstrual period.

**Chromosomal aberration:** alteration in the number or physical structure of chromosomes.

**Chromosome:** a DNA molecule that contains genes in linear order to which numerous proteins are bound.

**Codon:** a sequence of three adjacent nucleotides in an mRNA molecule, specifying either an amino acid or a stop signal in protein synthesis.

**Consanguinity:** degree of relationship between persons who descend from a common ancestor.

**Degenerate:** a feature of the genetic code in which an amino acid corresponds to more than one codon.

**Deletion:** loss of chromosomal material.

**Deoxyribonucleic acid (DNA):** a macromolecule usually composed of two polynucleotide chains in a double helix that is the carrier of genetic information in all cells.

**Dominant:** refers to an allele whose presence in a heterozygous genotype results in a phenotype characteristic of the allele.

**Down syndrome:** a chromosomal dysgenesis syndrome consisting of a variable constellation of abnormalities caused by triplication or translocation of chromosome 21. Affected individuals have some degree of mental retardation, characteristic facial features, and, often, heart defects and other health problems.

**Gene:** a region of DNA containing genetic information, which is usually transcribed into an RNA molecule that is processed and either functions directly or is translated into a polypeptide chain; the hereditary unit.

**Genomics:** systematic study of an organism's genome using large-scale DNA sequencing, gene-expression analysis, or computational methods.

**Germinal mutation:** a mutation that takes place in a reproductive cell.

**Hemizygous:** describes an individual who has only one member of a chromosome pair or chromosome segment rather than the usual two; refers in particular to X-linked genes in males who under usual circumstances have only one X chromosome.

**Heterozygous:** carrying dissimilar alleles of one or more genes; not homozygous.

**Homozygous:** having the same allele of a gene in homologous chromosomes.

**Inborn errors of metabolism:** a genetically determined biochemical disorder, usually in the form of an enzyme defect that produces a metabolic block.

**Inversion:** a structural aberration in a chromosome in which the order of several genes is reversed from the normal order.

**Klinefelter syndrome:** a disorder that occurs when an ovum with an extra X chromosome is fertilized by a sperm with a Y chromosome. This results in an XXY genotype male who is sterile.

**Locus:** the site or position of a particular gene on a chromosome.

**Mendelian genetics:** the mechanism of inheritance in which the statistical relations between the distribution of traits in successive generations result from three factors: (1) particulate hereditary determinants (genes), (2) random union of gametes, and (3) segregation of unchanged hereditary determinants in the reproductive cells.

**Messenger ribonucleic acid (mRNA):** an RNA molecule that is transcribed from a DNA sequence and translated into the amino acid sequence of a polypeptide.

**Mitochondrial chromosome:** a small circular chromosome found in each mitochondrion that encodes tRNA, rRNA, and proteins that are involved in oxidative phosphorylation and ATP generation.

**Monogenic:** of, relating to, or controlled by a single gene, especially by either of an allelic pair.

**Monosomy:** a condition in an otherwise diploid organism in which one member of a pair of chromosomes is missing.

**Mutation:** heritable alteration in a gene or chromosome; also, the process by which such an alteration happens.

**Nondisjunction:** failure of chromosomes to separate (disjoin) and move to opposite poles of the division spindle; the result is loss or gain of a chromosome.

**Pedigree analysis:** a diagram representing the familial relationships among relatives.

**Polygenic:** genetic disorder resulting from the combined action of alleles of more than one gene.

**Polysomy:** condition of a diploid cell or organism that has three or more copies of a particular chromosome.

**Recessive:** refers to an allele, or the corresponding phenotypic trait, that is expressed only in homozygotes.

**Ribosomal RNA (rRNA):** a type of RNA molecule that is a component of the ribosomal subunits.

**Sex chromosome:** a chromosome, such as the human X or Y, that plays a role in the determination of sex.

**Somatic mutation:** a mutation arising in a somatic cell.

**Transcription:** the process by which the information contained in a template strand of DNA is copied into a single-stranded RNA molecule of complementary base sequence.

**Transfer ribonucleic acids (tRNA):** a small RNA molecule that translates a codon into an amino acid in protein synthesis; it has a three-base sequence, called the anticodon, complementary to a specific codon in mRNA, and a site to which a specific amino acid is bound.

**Translation:** the process by which the amino acid sequence of a polypeptide is synthesized on a ribosome according to the nucleotide sequence of an mRNA molecule.

**Translocation:** a mutation results from an exchange of parts of two chromosomes.

**Trisomy:** a disorder in which a normally diploid organism has an extra copy of one of the chromosomes.

**Truncated protein:** a protein that does not achieve its full length or its proper form, and thus is missing some of the amino acid residues that are present in a normal protein. A truncated protein generally cannot perform the function for which it was intended because its structure is incapable of doing so.

**Turner syndrome:** a monosomy syndrome that results when an ovum lacking the X chromosome is fertilized by a sperm that contains an X chromosome. It may also occur when a genetically normal ovum is fertilized by a sperm lacking an X or Y chromosome. The result is an offspring with 22 pairs of autosomes and a single, unmatched X chromosome.

## Chapter Review Questions

1. The _____ encodes a few of the proteins for oxidative metabolism and all of the _____ used in translation of proteins within this organelle.

2. A change in DNA that could adversely affect the host that occurs after conception is termed a _____.

3. The three types of aneuploidy are _____, _____, and _____.

4. Autosomal recessive phenotypes are often associated with deficient activity of enzymes and, therefore, are termed _____.

5. Due to the presence of one X chromosome, males are said to be _____ for the mutant allele on that chromosome.

## Resources

American Academy of Pediatrics Committee on Genetics. Health Supervision for Children with Down Syndrome. *Pediatrics.* 107(2):442–449; 2001.

American College of Obstetricians and Gynecologists (ACOG). Screening for Fetal Chromosomal Abnormalities. *ACOG Practice Bulletin,* 77; January 2007.

Chiras, DD. *Human Biology,* 5th ed. Sudbury, MA: Jones and Bartlett; 2005.

Down Syndrome: March of Dimes. http://www.marchofdimes.com/pnhec/4439_1214.asp.

Fauci AS, Kasper DL, Braunwald E. et al. *Harrison's Principles of Internal Medicine,* 17th ed. http://www.accessmedicine.com; 2008.

Ferguson-Smith MA, et al. Cytogenetic Analysis. In: Rimoin DL, et al. (Eds.), *Emery and Rimoin's Principles and Practice of Medical Genetics,* 5th ed. Churchill Livingstone; 2007.

Friis RH, Sellers TA. *Epidemiology for Public Health Practice,* 3rd ed. Sudbury, MA: Jones and Bartlett; 2004.

Genetics Home Reference. http://ghr.nlm.nih.gov.

Genetics in the Physician Assistant's Practice. http://pa.nchpeg.org/.

Genomics and Its Impact on Science and Society: The Human Genome Project and Beyond. http://www.ornl.gov/sci/techresources/Human_Genome/publicat/primer 2001/4.shtml.

Hartl DL, Jones EW. *Genetics: Analysis of Genes and Genomes,* 6th ed. Sudbury, MA: Jones and Bartlett; 2005.

Hartl DL, Jones EW. *Essential Genetics: A Genomic Perspective,* 4th ed. Sudbury, MA: Jones and Bartlett; 2006.

Hook EB, Lindsjö A. Down Syndrome in Live Births by Single Year Maternal Age Interval in a Swedish Study: Comparison with Results from a New York State Study. *American Journal of Human Genetics.* 30:19–27; 1978.

Jameson JL, Kopp P. Principles of Human Genetics. In: Fauci AS, Braunwald E, Kasper DL, et al. (Eds.), *Harrison's Principles of Internal Medicine,* 17th ed. http://www.accessmedicine.com/content.aspx? aID= 2879424.

Jorde LB, Carey JC, Bamshad MJ, White RL. *Medical Genetics,* 3rd ed. St. Louis, MO: Mosby; 2006.

MedicineNet.com. http://www.medicinenet.com/script/main/hp.asp.

National Down Syndrome Society. http://www.ndss.org/index.php.

National Office of Public Health Genomics. http://www.cdc.gov/genomics/update/current.htm.

Nephrogenic Diabetes Insipidus Foundation. http://www.ndif.org/terms/18785-truncated_protein.

Pyeritz RE. Medical Genetics. In: Tierney LM Jr., McPhee SJ, Papadakis MA (Eds.), *Current Medical Diagnosis and Treatment,* 42nd ed. McGraw Hill Higher Education; 2003, pp. 1643–1666. http://www.accessmedicine.com/content.aspx? aID= 774551.

*Stedman's Online Medical Dictionary.* http://www.stedmans.com/.

Tierney LM Jr., McPhee SJ, Papadakis MA (Eds.). *Current Medical Diagnosis and Treatment,* 42nd ed. McGraw Hill Higher Education; 2003.

Westman JA. *Medical Genetics for the Modern Clinician.* Philadelphia, PA: Lippincott Williams & Wilkins; 2006.

# Chapter 2

# Diagnostic Techniques in Medical Genetics

## CHAPTER OBJECTIVES

✓ Review pedigree analysis and its associated terminology.
✓ Discuss the methodology and applications for cytogenetic studies.
✓ Explain fluorescence in situ hybridization.
✓ Describe DNA analysis and biochemical analysis.

Because hereditary disorders can affect different organ systems as well as people of all ages, it is important for healthcare providers to be familiar with genetic testing methodology. These tests range from taking a thorough family history that includes several familial generations (i.e., pedigree), to DNA sequencing, to hybridization with specific probes. While it is impractical to construct a detailed pedigree with every patient visit due to time constraints, it is important to know how to map out a pedigree in case there is some concern about a specific disease within a family.

## Family History

Clinicians are well trained in the importance of taking a good family history and should at the very least ask about the medical history of all first-degree relatives (parents, siblings, and offspring) and, if possible, more distant relatives. Pertinent information includes age, sex, ethnicity, general health status, major illnesses, and cause of death. Once this information is obtained, it can be further analyzed utilizing a pedigree diagram to identify mode of inheritance for a disease process.

## Pedigree Analysis

A pedigree is a diagram representing the familial relationships among relatives. It can be used to analyze Mendelian inheritance of certain traits. The symbols have been standardized, in that females are represented by circles and males by squares (**Figure 2-1**). A diamond is used if the sex is unknown. In the case of a miscarriage, a triangle is used. Colored or shaded symbols show persons with the phenotype of interest, whereas heterozygous carriers of recessive alleles are depicted with half-filled symbols.

A mating between a male and a female is indicated by a single horizontal line that is then connected vertically with a second horizontal line below that connects the symbols for their offspring. Mating between related (**consanguineous**) individuals is indicated

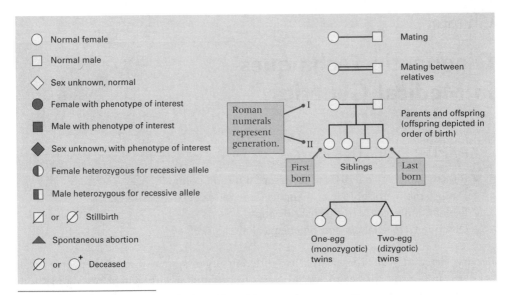

**Figure 2-1** Conventional symbols used in depicting human pedigrees.
*Source:* Bennett R, French K, Resta R, Doyle D. Standardized Human Pedigree Nomenclature: Update and Assessment of the Recommendations of the National Society of Genetic Counselors. *Journal of Genetic Counseling.* 17:424–433;2008. ©National Society of Genetic Counselors, Inc. 2008.

with a double horizontal line. The offspring, called **sibs** or **siblings**, are represented from left to right in order of birth; each row corresponds to a generation that is labeled with a Roman numeral.

**Figure 2-2** shows an example of a pedigree for a family in which some members have Huntington's disease (see Chapter 4). Within any generation, the individuals are numbered consecutively from left to right. The pedigree starts with the woman I-1 and the man is I-2. The man has Huntington's disease, as indicated by the shaded symbol. Because this disease is due to a dominant mutation, all affected individuals have the heterozygous genotype *HD hd*, whereas nonaffected people have the homozygous normal genotype *hd*

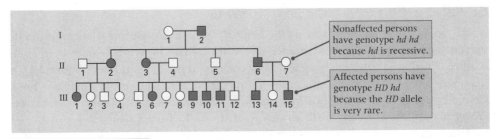

**Figure 2-2** Pedigree of a human family showing the inheritance of the gene for Huntington's disease. Females and males are represented by circles and squares. Shaded symbols indicate people affected with the disease.

*hd*. The disease has complete **penetrance**, which means the trait is expressed in 100% of persons with that genotype.

For example, in the case of a rare dominant allele with complete penetrance, the following characteristics are observed:

1. Females and males are affected equally.

2. Affected offspring typically have one affected parent, with the same likelihood ratio of the affected parent being the mother or the father.

3. Approximately 50% the siblings with the same parents are affected.

An example of a pedigree for a homozygous recessive allele is albinism (**Figure 2-3**). In comparison, inheriting a rare recessive allele with complete penetrance, would yield the following observed characteristics:

1. Females and males are affected equally.

2. Affected individuals would *not* have affected offspring.

3. Affected individuals typically have *no* affected parents.

4. Parents of those affected may be related.

5. Approximately 25% of siblings with the same parents are affected.

> In the case of inheritance of a rare recessive trait, the mates of homozygous affected persons are usually homozygous for the normal allele, so all of the offspring will be heterozygous and not affected. Because it is more likely that a person will inherit only one copy of a rare mutant allele rather than two copies, heterozygous carriers of

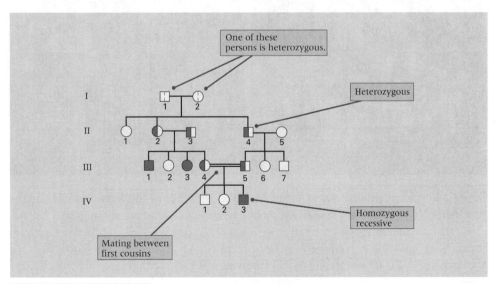

**Figure 2-3** Pedigree of albinism. With recessive inheritance, affected persons (filled symbols) often have unaffected parents. The double horizontal line indicates a mating between relatives—in this case, first cousins.

mutant alleles are more common than homozygous affected individuals. Therefore, most homozygous recessive genotypes result from mating between heterozygous carriers in which each offspring has a 25% chance of being affected. This can especially occur if parents of affected individuals are related. (Hartl and Jones, 2005)

A rare recessive allele (i.e., albinism) is more likely to be expressed when mating between related heterozygous individuals occurs (Figure 2-3). The offspring resulting from this mating has a 25% chance of inheriting the homozygous recessive allele and will express the albino trait.

## Cytogenetic Studies

Cytogenetics is the study of chromosomes utilizing light microscopy. Chromosomal analysis is done by growing human cells in tissue culture, chemically inhibiting mitosis, staining, observing, photographing, sorting, and counting the chromosomes. Samples can be obtained from peripheral blood, amniotic fluid, trophoblastic cells from the chorionic villus, bone marrow, and cultured fibroblasts (usually obtained from a skin biopsy). In a **karyotype**, the chromosomes are rearranged systematically in pairs, from longest to shortest, and numbered from 1 (the longest) through 22 to represent the autosomes (**Figure 2-4**). The sex chromosomes are usually set off at the bottom right. The karyotype

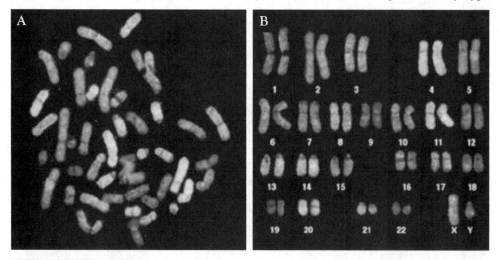

**Figure 2-4** Human chromosome painting, in which each pair of chromosomes is labeled by hybridization with a different fluorescent probe. (A) Metaphase spread showing the chromosomes in a random arrangement as they were squashed onto the slide. (B) A karyotype, in which the chromosomes have been grouped in pairs and arranged in conventional order. Chromosomes 1–20 are arranged in order of decreasing size, but for historical reasons, chromosome 21 precedes chromosome 22, even though chromosome 21 is smaller.
*Source:* Courtesy of Johannes Wienberg, Ludwig-Macimillians-University, and Thomas Ried, National Institutes of Health.

of a normal human female has a pair of X chromosomes instead of an X and a Y. **Chromosome painting**, as shown in Figure 2-4, helps to identify pairs of homologous chromosomes. The different colors are "painted" on each chromosome by hybridization with DNA strands labeled with different fluorescent dyes.

Another karyotype is shown in **Figure 2-5** with chromosome banding. These chromosomes have been treated with Giemsa stain, which causes chromosomes to exhibit transverse bands (G-bands) that are specific for each pair of homologs. These bands allow smaller segments of each chromosome arm to be identified. In addition to allowing the identification of autosomes and sex chromosomes, chromosomal abnormalities can be identified through this technique.

## Fluorescence in Situ Hybridization

Chromosome staining and painting provides a way to visualize banding patterns and pairs of homologous chromosomes. However, this interpretation can be rather difficult given that a "standard" karyotype reveals approximately 400 to 500 bands per set of haploid chromosomes. The development of fluorescence in situ hybridization (FISH) has made it easier to visualize and map chromosomal (gene) abnormalities.

"Fluorescent means emitting light that comes from a reaction within the emitter and "in situ" refers to the fact that this technique is done with the chromosomes, cells or tissue in place (in situ) on a microscope slide" (MedicineNet, 2010). A short sequence of nucleic

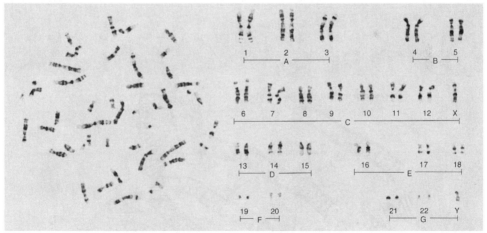

**(A)** Photograph of metaphase chromosomes    **(B)** Karyotype

**Figure 2-5** A karyotype of a normal human male. Blood cells arrested in metaphase were stained with Giemsa and photographed with a microscope. (A) The chromosomes as seen in the cell by microscopy. (B) The chromosomes have been cut out of the photograph and paired with their homologs.
*Source:* Courtesy of Patricia A. Jacobs, Wessex Regional Genetics Laboratory, Salisbury District Hospital.

acid that matches a portion of the gene in question is labeled with a fluorescent dye and is referred to as a **probe**. The probe is then allowed to hybridize to suitably prepared cells or histological sections; hybrids are formed with complementary sequences of nucleic acids in a chromosome (**Figure 2-6**). Through nucleic acid hybridization, the degree of sequence identity can be determined and specific sequences detected and located on a specific chromosome (MedicineNet, 2010). This technique is frequently used to look for localization of genes on specific chromosomes.

## INDICATIONS FOR CYTOGENETIC ANALYSIS

- Malformations associated with a particular syndrome or aberration
- Serious mental or physical developmental problems
- Maldefined genitalia (internal or external)
- Primary amenorrhea or delayed pubertal development
- Males with learning or behavioral disorders who are taller than expected
- Malignant or premalignant disease
- Parents of a patient with a chromosome translocation
- Parents of a patient with a suspected syndrome
- Couples with a history of multiple spontaneous abortions of unknown cause
- Infertility not caused by obstetric or urogenital problems
- Prenatal diagnosis

*Source:* Reproduced from Pyeritz RE. Medical Genetics. In Tierney L, et al. *Current Medical Diagnosis & Treatment*, 42nd ed. 2003.

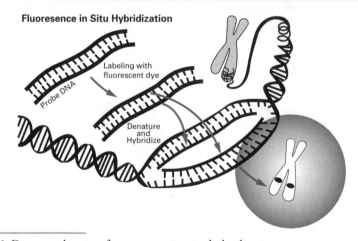

**Figure 2-6** Diagram showing fluorescence in situ hybridization.
*Source:* Courtesy of Fluorescence In Situ (FISH) National Genome Research Institute, National Institutes of Health. Available at http://www.genome.gov/10000206. Accessed January 16, 2010.

## DNA Analysis

Molecular genetics involves understanding the expression of genes by studying DNA sequences of chromosomes. Once a particular gene is shown to be defective in a given disease, the nature of the mutation can be elucidated by sequencing the nucleotides and comparing with that of a normal allele. Molecular testing is available for more than 1000 hereditary conditions and has had a significant impact on the diagnosis of Mendelian disorders.

Similar to the use of specific probes in a FISH analysis of chromosomal abnormalities, probes are used to identify specific genes that may be mutated in a certain hereditary disease. The probe may be a piece of the actual gene, a sequence close to the gene, or just a few nucleotides at the actual mutation. The closer the probe is to the actual mutation, the more accurate and the more useful the information. When even a minute amount of DNA from a patient (e.g., from a few leukocytes, buccal mucosal cells, or hair bulbs) is combined with the primers in a reaction mixture that replicates DNA—and after several dozen replication cycles are then performed via a process called **polymerase chain reaction (PCR)**—the region of DNA between the primers will be amplified exponentially. For example, the presence of early HIV infection can be detected after PCR amplification of a portion of the viral genome.

### EXAMPLE INDICATIONS FOR DNA ANALYSIS

- Pre-symptomatic detection of Huntington's disease or adult polycystic kidney disease
- Screening for cystic fibrosis and thalassemias
- Screening for X-linked conditions such as Duchenne muscular dystrophy and hemophilia A and B
- Screening for familial polyposis coli

*Source:* Reproduced from Pyeritz RE. Medical Genetics. In Tierney et al. *Current Medical Diagnosis and Treatment*, 42nd ed. 2003.

## Biochemical Analysis

The primary goal of biochemical testing is to determine whether certain proteins are present or absent as well as to identify their characteristics and effectiveness in vitro. This kind of analysis is used to look for enzymatic defects, as these important catalysts are made of protein. For example, **phenylketonuria (PKU)** is an inherited disorder caused by the absence of or a defect in the enzyme **phenylalanine hydroxylase (PAH)**. In the absence of PAH, the amino acid phenylalanine accumulates and can lead to severe mental retardation. If this deficiency is diagnosed early in life, however, children can be placed on low-phenylalanine diets and mental retardation avoided. Based on this knowledge, all babies in the United States are screened for PKU.

Another disease process associated with a defective protein is **cystic fibrosis (CF)**. In this disease, a mutation in the **CFTR gene** disrupts chloride and water transport across membranes. The end result is production of thick and sticky mucus that obstructs the airways in the lungs and the ducts in the pancreas. In addition to breathing difficulty, people with CF have problems with nutrient digestion because the buildup of mucus prevents pancreatic digestive enzymes from reaching the intestine.

Both PKU and CF are examples of **inborn errors of metabolism**, which refers to an inherited defect in one or more enzymes. Currently, the state of Georgia screens newborns for 24 metabolic disorders plus sickle cell anemia. Not all states test for all of the same disorders in their screening of infants, however, and in some cases parents can refuse to have the tests done. For a more detailed listing and description of inborn errors of metabolism, refer to the United States National Newborn Screening Status Report at http://genes-r-us.uthscsa.edu/nbsdisorders.pdf.

## Chapter Summary

- A good family history should at the very least ask about the medical history of all first-degree relatives (parents, siblings, and offspring) and, if possible, more distant relatives.
- A pedigree can be used to analyze Mendelian inheritance of certain traits.
- Cytogenetics is the study of chromosomes utilizing light microscopy.
- Once a particular gene is shown to be defective in a given disease, the nature of the mutation can be elucidated by sequencing the nucleotides and comparing this sequence with that of a normal allele.
- The primary goal of biochemical testing is to determine whether certain proteins are present or absent as well as to identify their characteristics and effectiveness in vitro.

## Key Terms

**CFTR gene:** a gene that codes for a protein involved in chloride and water transport across membranes. In patients with cystic fibrosis, a mutation in this gene disrupts chloride and water transport across membranes. The end result is production of thick and sticky mucus that obstructs the airways in the lungs and the ducts in the pancreas.

**Chromosome painting:** use of differentially labeled, chromosome-specific DNA strands for hybridization with chromosomes to label each chromosome with a different color.

**Consanguineous:** mating between related individuals.

**Cystic fibrosis:** a congenital metabolic disorder, inherited as an autosomal recessive trait, in which secretions of exocrine glands are abnormal. Excessively viscid mucus causes obstruction of passageways (including pancreatic and bile ducts, intestines, and bronchi), and the sodium and chloride content of sweat are increased throughout the patient's life

**Inborn error of metabolism:** a genetically determined biochemical disorder, usually in the form of an enzyme defect that produces a metabolic block.

**Karyotype:** the chromosome complement of a cell or organism; often represented by an arrangement of metaphase chromosomes according to their lengths and the positions of their centromeres.

**Penetrance:** the proportion of organisms having a particular genotype that actually express the corresponding phenotype. If the phenotype is always expressed, penetrance is complete; otherwise, it is incomplete.

**Phenylalanine hydroxylase (PAH):** the enzyme that converts phenylalanine to tyrosine and that is defective in phenylketonuria.

**Phenylketonuria (PKU):** a hereditary human condition resulting from inability to convert phenylalanine into tyrosine. It causes severe mental retardation unless treated in infancy and childhood by a low-phenylalanine diet.

**Polymerase chain reaction (PCR):** repeated cycles of DNA denaturation, renaturation with primer oligonucleotide sequences, and replication, resulting in exponential growth in the number of copies of the DNA sequence located between the primers.

**Probe:** a labeled DNA or RNA molecule used in DNA-RNA or DNA-DNA hybridization assays.

**Sibling (sib):** a brother or sister, each having the same parents.

## Chapter Review Questions

1. Mating between related individuals, also known as _____, is indicated with a double horizontal line in a pedigree diagram.

2. Siblings of individuals who carry the recessive gene for albinism have a _____ percent chance of inheriting and being affected by this trait.

3. In a _____, the chromosomes are rearranged systematically in pairs, from longest to shortest, and numbered from 1 (the longest) through 22.

4. _____ with a fluorescent probe is one method used to assess the degree of sequence identity as well as detect and locate specific sequences on a specific chromosome.

5. In the absence of _____, the amino acid phenylalanine accumulates and can lead to severe mental retardation.

## Resources

*The American Heritage Dictionary of the English Language,* 4th ed. Boston: Houghton Mifflin; 2006.

Bennett RL, French KS, Resta RG, Doyle DL. Standardized Human Pedigree Nomenclature: Update and Assessment of the Recommendations of the National Society of Genetic Counselors. *Journal of Genetic Counseling.* 17:424–433; 2008.

Georgia Department of Human Resources. Newborn Screening for Metabolic and Sickle Cell Disorders Program. http://health.state.ga.us/programs/nsmscd/descriptions.asp.

Hartl, DL, Jones EW. *Genetics: Analysis of Genes and Genomes,* 6th ed. Sudbury, MA: Jones and Bartlett; 2005.

Hartl, DL, Jones EW. *Essential Genetics: A Genomic Perspective,* 4th ed. Sudbury, MA: Jones and Bartlett; 2006.

MedicineNet, Inc. Definition of Fluorescent in Situ Hybridization. Available at http://www.medterms.com/script/main/art.asp?articlekey=3486. Accessed January 27, 2010.

National Newborn Screening and Genetics Resource Center. http://genes-r-us.uthscsa.edu/.

Pyeritz RE. Medical Genetics. In: Tierney LM Jr., McPhee SJ, Papadakis MA (Eds.), *Current Medical Diagnosis and Treatment,* 42nd ed. New York: McGraw-Hill; 2003, pp. 1643–1666.

*Stedman's Online Medical Dictionary.* http://www.stedmans.com/.

# Chapter 3

# Development and Teratogenesis

## CHAPTER OBJECTIVES

✓ Review basic embryology.
✓ Understand the etiology and distribution of congenital anomalies.
✓ Define teratogenesis and describe the three main principles underlying this process.
✓ Describe major defects involved with examples of teratogens.

During fertilization, sperm come into contact with the plasma membrane of the oocyte. This interaction triggers meiotic division, which results in the formation of the ovum or egg. Once the sperm enters the ovum, the nuclei combine to form a **zygote** that contains 46 chromosomes. The next step is the first mitotic division—one of many billions of such divisions that will occur during human growth and development. Throughout this process, a clear distinction is made between weeks of pregnancy and weeks of development. Pregnancy starts with the first day of the last menstrual period, whereas development starts at fertilization (usually two weeks after the last menstrual period).

## Embryonic Development

Human development consists of three stages, labeled as pre-embryonic, embryonic, and fetal. The pre-embryonic stage includes all of the changes that occur from fertilization to the time just after an embryo becomes implanted in the uterine wall. During this phase, the zygote undergoes rapid cellular division and is converted into a solid ball of cells called a **morula** (**Figure 3-1**). Three to four days after fertilization, repeated cell cleavages yield a total of 16 to 32 cells. By this time, the morula has reached the uterus; during the next three to four days, it floats in the intrauterine fluid as more cell divisions occur.

Fluid soon begins to accumulate in the morula and creates a hollow sphere of cells called a **blastocyst**. This stage consists of a clump of cells, the **inner cell mass** (ICM), which will eventually become the **embryo**, and a ring of flattened cells, the **trophoblast**. The trophoblast will further develop into the embryonic portion of the **placenta** that supplies nutrients to and removes wastes from the embryo.

## Implantation

The blastocyst attaches to the uterine wall six or seven days after fertilization. For the next few weeks, cells of the trophoblast secrete enzymes that digest the adjacent endometrial cells so that the embryo can obtain nourishment. However, if the endometrium is not

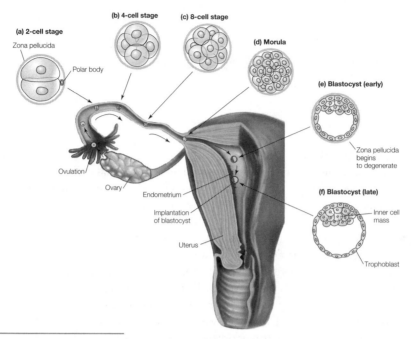

**Figure 3-1** Formation of the morula and blastocyst during pre-embryonic development.

ready for any reason, the blastocyst cannot implant. This implantation can be prevented by the presence of an endometrial infection, an intrauterine device, or use of a **morning after pill**. Blastocysts may also fail to implant if their cells contain certain genetic mutations. Unimplanted blastocysts are absorbed (through a process called phagocytosis) by the endometrium or expelled during menstruation.

If implantation does occur, by day 14 the uterine endometrium grows over the blastocyst, enclosing it and walling it off from the rest of the uterine cavity. Endometrial cells respond to the attached blastocyst by producing **paracrines**, such as prostaglandins, that promote local changes in the endometrial tissue. These changes include increased development of uterine blood vessels, which helps to ensure delivery of oxygen and other nutrients to the area. Soon after this stage, the maternal (endometrium) and embryonic (trophoblast) tissues combine to form the placenta.

Early in the development of the placenta, a layer of cells separates from the ICM to form the **amnion** and a small cavity forms between the ICM and amnion. This amniotic cavity fills with amniotic fluid that, in addition to providing nutrients, acts like a "shock absorber" to protect the fetus from injury during development. After the amnion is formed, the cells of the ICM differentiate to create three distinct germ layers: the **ectoderm**, the **mesoderm**, and the **endoderm**. Known as the primary germ layers, their formation marks the beginning of embryonic development and will give rise to the organs by a process called **organogenesis**. **Table 3-1** shows the organs that form from each layer.

Table 3-1    **Organs and Tissues Associated with Embryonic Germ Layers**

| Endoderm | Mesoderm | Ectoderm |
| --- | --- | --- |
| Lining of digestive system | Dermis | Epidermis |
| Lining of respiratory system | All muscles of the body | Hair, nails, sweat glands |
| Urethra and urinary bladder | Cartilage | Brain and spinal cord |
| Gallbladder | Bone | Cranial and spinal nerves |
| Liver and pancreas | Blood | Retina, lens, and cornea of eye |
| Thyroid gland | All other connective tissue | Inner ear |
| Parathyroid gland | Blood vessels | Epithelium of nose, mouth, and anus |
| Thymus | Reproductive organs | |
| Kidneys | Enamel of teeth | |

*Source:* Adapted from Chiras DD. *Human Biology*, 5th ed. 2005.

The formation of the central nervous system (spinal cord, brain) is one of the first steps of organogenesis. Early in embryonic development, the ectoderm located along the back of the embryo folds inward. This creates a long trench—the neural groove that runs the length of the back surface of the embryo. During the next few weeks, this neural groove deepens and eventually closes off, thereby creating the neural tube. The walls of the neural tube thicken to form the spinal cord. In the head region, the neural tube expands to form the brain. The spinal and cranial nerves develop from small aggregations of ectodermal cells (the neural crest) that are found on either side of the neural tube. These cells eventually develop into axons that grow throughout the body and attach to organs, muscle, bone, and skin. The ectoderm is also the precursor for the epidermis.

The mesoderm is the middle germ layer, which gives rise to body tissues such as muscle, cartilage, bone, and dermis. The endoderm contributes to the formation of a large pouch under the embryo called the **yolk sac**. The uppermost part of the yolk sac develops into the lining of the intestinal tract. It also gives rise to blood cells and primitive germ cells. During organogenesis, the germ cells migrate from the wall of the yolk sac to the developing testes or ovaries. These cells eventually become spermatogonia or oogonia.

Fetal development involves ongoing organ development and growth as well as changes in body proportions. It begins in the eighth week of pregnancy and ends at **parturition** (birth). The fetus grows rapidly during this period, increasing in length from approximately 2.5 centimeters to 35 to 50 centimeters and increasing in weight from 1 gram to 3000 to 4000 grams. The fetus also becomes more humanlike in physical appearance with each month of gestation. The organ development that started during the embryonic stage is completed during the fetal stage.

## Congenital Abnormalities

It has been estimated that 31% of all successful fertilizations end in miscarriage or spontaneous abortion. Approximately 66% of these miscarriages occur before a woman is even aware that she is pregnant. This high frequency is thought to reflect how nature deals with defective embryos. This system of dealing with abnormalities is not perfect, however, as many children are born each year with birth defects. Between 10% and 12% of all newborns have some kind of birth defect, ranging from a minor biochemical problem to some sort of gross physical deformity. Such defects may be caused by a variety of biological, chemical, and physical agents. Some contributors to these congenital abnormalities include mutant genes, chromosomal defects, and multifactorial components. Unfortunately, the largest cause of these defects is of unknown etiology.

Teratology is the study of abnormal development (**Table 3-2**). Teratogens include anything capable of disrupting embryonic or fetal development and producing malformations (i.e., birth defects). A host of chemical, physical, and biological agents may cause developmental anomalies (**Tables 3-3 and 3-4**). Most complex developmental abnormalities affecting several organ systems result from injuries inflicted from the time of implantation of the blastocyst through early organogenesis. "The stage of embryonic development most susceptible to teratogenesis is during the formation of primordial organ systems. Many major defects probably result from faulty gene activity or the deleterious effects of exogenous toxins on the embryo at this time" (Rubin, 2001).

The critical period for teratogenic effects is between 3 and 16 weeks of gestation. Three major factors that affect the likelihood and extent of teratogenesis are dosage, time of exposure, and genotype of the embryo. Because organ systems develop at different times, the timing of exposure determines which systems are affected by a given agent (**Figure 3-2**). During its critical development period, an organ is vulnerable to toxins, viruses, and genetic abnormalities. Any alteration of normal development may cause birth defects. The central nervous system begins to develop during the third week of pregnancy, whereas the teeth, palate, and genitalia do not begin to form until about the sixth or seventh week of pregnancy. Therefore, exposure to some teratogen during the seventh week of pregnancy

Table 3-2 **Principles of Teratology**

1. Susceptibility to teratogens is variable.

2. Susceptibility to teratogens is specific for each developmental stage.

3. The mechanism of teratogenesis is specific for each teratogen.

4. Teratogenesis is dose dependent.

5. Teratogens produce death, growth retardation, malformation, or functional impairment.

*Source:* Data from Rubin E. *Essential Pathology*, 3rd ed. 2001.

Table 3-3  **Types of Teratogens**

| | |
|---|---|
| Pharmacological | Thalidomide<br>Diethylstilbesterol<br>Retinoic acid |
| Infectious agents | *Toxoplasma gondii*<br>Rubella<br>Cytomegalovirus<br>Herpes<br>Congenital syphilis |
| Industrial agents | Lead<br>Mercury<br>Pesticides/herbicides |
| Recreational | Alcohol<br>Tobacco<br>Cocaine |

Table 3-4  **Common Drugs That Are Teratogenic or Fetotoxic**

| | | |
|---|---|---|
| ACE inhibitors | Diethylstilbesterol | Progestins |
| Alcohol | Disulfiram | Radioiodine |
| Amandatine | Ergotamine | Reserpine |
| Androgens | Estrogens | Ribavirin |
| Anticonvulsants | Griseofulvin | Sulfonamides |
| Aspirin and other salicylates (third trimester) | Hypoglycemics, oral (older drugs) | SSRIs |
| Benzodiazepines | Isotretinoin | Tetracycline (third trimester) |
| Carbarsone | Lithium | Thalidomide |
| Chloramphenicol (third trimester) | Methotrexate | Tobacco smoking |
| Cyclophosphamide | NSAIDs (third trimester) | Trimethoprim (third trimester) |
| Diazoxide | Opioids (prolonged use) | Warfarin (Coumadin) and other anticoagulants |

ACE: angiotensin-converting enzyme; NSAIDs: nonsteroidal anti-inflammatory drugs; SSRIs: selective serotonin reuptake inhibitors.
*Source*: Crombleholme WR. Chapter 19: Obstetrics & Obstetric Disorders. McPhee SJ, Papadakis MA, Tierney LM, Jr. *Current Medical Diagnosis & Treatment*, 48th ed; 2009. http://www.accessmedicine.com/content.aspx?aID=9353. Copyright © The McGraw-Hill Companies, Inc. All rights reserved.

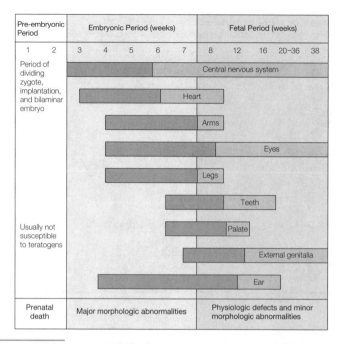

**Figure 3-2** Human development is divided into three stages: pre-embryonic, embryonic, and fetal. Organogenesis occurs during the embryonic stage. Each bar indicates when an organ system develops. The dark-shaded area indicates the periods most sensitive to teratogenic agents.

may affect the genitalia, palate, or teeth, but have little effect on the central nervous system because it has entered a less sensitive phase of development.

## Thalidomide

Thalidomide is used today to treat illnesses such as multiple myeloma, erythema nodosum leprosum, HIV wasting, and aphthous ulcers. It was originally developed in the 1950s for the treatment of pregnancy-associated morning sickness, but was withdrawn from the market due to the tragic consequences of its teratogenicity, which included stunted limb growth in affected fetuses. This drug was given to pregnant women to prevent morning sickness between weeks 4 and 10 of pregnancy, which is the critical period for limb formation. Among babies who survived, birth defects included deafness, blindness, disfigurement, cleft palate, and many other internal disabilities. However, the disabilities most closely associated with thalidomide involved defective development of arms or legs, or both, so that the hands and feet were attached close to the body, resembling the flippers of a seal (**phocomelia**; see **Figure 3-3**).

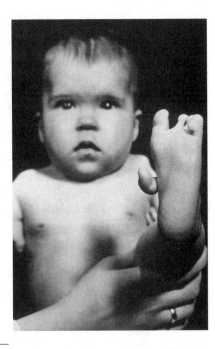

**Figure 3-3** Baby with malformed limbs due to in utero thalidomide exposure.
*Source:* © National Cancer Institute/Photo Researchers, Inc.

> The numbers vary from source to source as no proper census was ever taken, but it has been claimed that there were between ten and twenty thousand babies born disabled as a consequence of thalidomide. There are approximately 5,000 survivors alive today around the world. (Thalidomide Victims Association of Canada, 2010)

The number of babies who were miscarried or stillborn as a consequence of thalidomide has never been counted.

## TORCH Complex

A complex of similar signs and symptoms produced by fetal or neonatal infection with a variety of microorganisms is referred to as TORCH. This collection of infectious organisms includes *Toxoplasma* (T), rubella (R), cytomegalovirus (C), and herpes simplex virus (H); the letter "O" in the acronym represents "others." Children infected in utero with any of these agents have very similar symptoms.

Asymptomatic toxoplasmosis is common, with 25% of women in their reproductive years exhibiting antibodies to this organism. However, intrauterine *Toxoplasma* infection occurs in only 0.1% of all pregnancies.

Early in the 1960s, an epidemic of rubella occurred over a period of approximately two years; 20,000 children developed congenital rubella syndrome, and there were 30,000 still-births from this infection. "Rubella syndrome, or congenital rubella, is characterized by rash at birth, low birth weight, small head size, heart abnormalities (i.e., patent ductus arteriosis), visual problems (i.e., cataracts), and bulging fontanelle" (AllRefer.com, 2010). Fortunately, the introduction of the rubella vaccine in the United States has virtually eliminated congenital rubella.

"Cytomegalovirus (CMV) is a virus found around the world. It is related to the viruses that cause chickenpox and infectious mononucleosis Once CMV is in a person's body, it stays there for life" (Medline Plus, 2010). Approximately 66% of childbearing-age women test positive for CMV immunoglobulin G, and as many as 2% of newborns in the United States are congenitally infected with this virus. Newborns who survive are at increased risk for hearing loss and mental retardation. "However, only 3% of newborns infected with CMV during pregnancy experience problems from the virus. Most are born healthy or with only mild CMV symptoms" (FamilyDoctor.org, 2010).

Clinical and pathological findings in the symptomatic newborn with TORCH complex vary. Only a few present with multisystem disease and the entire spectrum of abnormalities. Lesions of the brain represent the most serious pathological changes in TORCH-infected children. Acute encephalitis is associated with foci of necrosis. **Microcephaly**, **hydrocephalus**, and abnormally shaped gyri and sulci are frequently observed. "Severe brain damage is reflected in psychomotor retardation, neurologic defects, and seizures" (Rubin, 2001). As mentioned earlier, ocular defects are prominent in children infected with rubella, with more than two thirds of these patients presenting with cataracts. In addition, congenital rubella often leads to cardiac anomalies, such as patent ductus arteriosus and various septal defects.

## Fetal Alcohol Syndrome

Ethyl alcohol (also known simply as alcohol) is one of the most potent teratogens known. Its use during pregnancy varies by population. A safe threshold dose for alcohol use during pregnancy has never been established (Crombleholme, 2007). Fetal alcohol syndrome comprises a complex of abnormalities caused by maternal consumption of alcohol and includes growth retardation, central nervous system dysfunction, and characteristic facial dysmorphology. Because not all children adversely affected by maternal alcohol abuse exhibit the entire spectrum of abnormalities, the term **fetal alcohol effect** is also used to describe this condition.

Children with fetal alcohol effect have milder degrees of mental deficiency and emotional disorders; this outcome is more common than the full fetal alcohol syndrome scenario. The minimum amount of alcohol that results in fetal injury is not well established, but children afflicted with fetal alcohol syndrome are usually the offspring of mothers with chronic alcoholism. Characteristic features associated with this syndrome are outlined in **Table 3-5**.

## Table 3-5   Characteristic Features Associated with Fetal Alcohol Syndrome

Behavior disturbances

Brain defects

Cardiac defects

Spinal defects

Craniofacial anomalies

 Absent or hypoplastic philtrum

 Broad upper lip

 Flattened nasal bridge

 Hypoplastic upper lip vermilion

 Micrognathia

 Microphthalmia

 Short nose

 Short palpebral tissues

*Source:* Cunningham FG, Leveno KL, Bloom SL, Hauth JC, Gilstrap LC III, Wenstrom KD, Chapter 14: Teratology, Drugs, and Other Medications. Cunningham FG, Leveno KL, Bloom SL, Hauth JC, Gilstrap LC III, Wenstrom KD. *Williams Obstetrics*, 22nd ed; 2009. Copyright © The McGraw-Hill Companies, Inc. All rights reserved.

It has been reported that 20% of children with fetal alcohol syndrome have IQs lower than 70, and 40% of the children have IQs between 70 and 85. (Normal IQ values are in the vicinity of 100.) The affected child may have congenital heart and joint defects as well as demonstrate failure to thrive and persistent irritability during the early years of life. These problems are followed by developmental delay, growth deficiency, and poor coordination. Other co-morbid conditions include mental retardation, attention-deficit/hyperactivity disorder, learning disorders, sensory impairment, cerebral palsy, and epilepsy.

## Tobacco

Cigarette smoke contains a number of potential teratogens, including nicotine, cotinine, cyanide, thiocyanate, carbon monoxide, cadmium, lead, and various hydrocarbons. In addition to being fetotoxic, many of these substances have vasoactive effects that reduce oxygen levels. A well-documented reproductive outcome related to smoking is a direct dose-response reduction in fetal growth. Newborns of mothers who smoke weigh, on average, 200 g less than newborns of nonsmoking mothers, and heavy smoking results in more severe weight reduction. Smoking doubles the risk of low birth weight, and increases the risk of a small-for-gestational age newborn by 2.5-fold. Women who stop smoking early in pregnancy generally have neonates with normal birth weights. Smoking also may cause a slightly increased incidence of subfertility, spontaneous abortion, placenta previa and abruption, and preterm delivery.

## Cocaine

Cocaine is currently one of the most widely abused drugs in the United States. This central nervous system stimulant exerts its effects through sympathomimetic action via dopamine. Cocaine is a highly effective topical anesthetic and local vasoconstrictor, and most of the adverse outcomes noted in offspring associated with pregnant women's use of cocaine result from the drug's vasoconstrictive and hypertensive effects. Maternal complications include myocardial infarction, arrhythmias, aortic rupture, stroke, seizure, bowel ischemia, and sudden death. Placental abruption is the most frequently cited cocaine-related pregnancy complication in cocaine abusers: Its incidence is fourfold greater in users than in nonusers.

The risk of vascular disruption within the embryo, fetus, or placenta is highest after the first trimester of pregnancy, and likely accounts for the increased incidence of stillbirth. A number of cocaine-related congenital anomalies resulting from vascular disruption have been described, including skull defects, cutis aplasia, **porencephaly**, subependymal and periventricular cysts, ileal atresia, cardiac anomalies, and visceral infarcts. Because few reports address dosage or total fetal exposure during pregnancy, it is difficult to estimate the precise fetal risk associated with antenatal cocaine use.

## Vitamin A

Beta-carotene is a precursor of vitamin A that is found in fruits and vegetables; it has not been shown to cause birth defects. Many foods contain the fat-soluble vitamin A, but animal liver contains the highest amounts. Excessive dietary intake of vitamin A has been associated with teratogenicity in humans. Therefore, caution must be used to avoid unnecessary supplementation of women of childbearing age.

Some vitamin A isomers are used for dermatological disorders because they stimulate epithelial cell differentiation. Isotretinoin, which is 13-*cis*-retinoic acid, is effective for treatment of cystic acne. It is also considered to be one of the most potent teratogens in widespread use. First-trimester exposure to this isomer is associated with a high rate of fetal loss, and the 26-fold increased malformation rate in survivors is similar to that observed among children exposed to thalidomide in utero. Abnormalities have been described only with first-trimester use of isotretinoin, however. Because isotretinoin is rapidly cleared from the body (its mean serum half-life is 12 hours), anomalies are not increased in women who discontinue therapy with this drug before conception.

Although any organ system can be affected by isotretinoin exposure, malformations typically involve the cranium and face, heart, central nervous system, and thymus. These defects frequently appear in conjunction with agenesis of the external ear canal. Other defects include cleft palate and maldevelopment of the facial bones and cranium. The most frequently noted cardiac anomalies are outflow tract defects, and hydrocephalus is the most common central nervous system defect.

## Diethylstilbestrol

From 1940 to 1971, between 2 million and 10 million pregnant women took diethylstilbesterol (DES) to "support" high-risk pregnancies. This drug later was shown to have no beneficial effects, and its use for this purpose was abandoned. In 1971, however, it was reported that eight women who had prenatal exposure to DES had developed vaginal clear-cell adenocarcinoma. Subsequent studies showed that the absolute cancer risk in prenatally exposed women is substantially increased, to about 1 per 1000. Malignancy is not dose related, and there is no relationship between the location of the tumor and the timing of exposure.

In the years since the first reports of a DES–cancer link surfaced, researchers have shown that DES produces both structural and functional abnormalities. Because DES interrupts the transition of cells within the developing vagina/cervix in as many as half of exposed female fetuses, DES-exposed women have a twofold increase in vaginal and cervical intraepithelial neoplasia. One fourth of exposed females have structural abnormalities of the cervix or vagina; the embryological mechanism underlying these defects is unknown. The most commonly reported abnormalities include a hypoplastic, T-shaped uterine cavity; cervical collars;, hoods, septa, and coxcombs; and "withered" fallopian tubes. Affected women are at increased risk for poor pregnancy outcomes related to uterine malformations, decreased endometrial thickness, and reduced uterine perfusion. Exposed male fetuses have normal sexual function and fertility, but are at increased risk for epididymal cysts, microphallus, cryptorchidism, testicular hypoplasia, and hypospadias.

## Chapter Summary

- Human development proceeds through three stages: pre-embryonic, embryonic, and fetal.

- The ectoderm, mesoderm, and endoderm are the primary germ layers; their formation marks the beginning of embryonic development. As the embryo develops, these layers give rise to the organs by a process called organogenesis.

- An estimated 31% of all successful fertilizations end in miscarriage or spontaneous abortion; 66% of these miscarriages occur before a woman is even aware that she is pregnant.

- Teratology is the study of abnormal development; teratogens include anything capable of disrupting embryonic or fetal development and producing malformations.

- The critical period for teratogenic effects is between 3 and 16 weeks of gestation.

- Three factors known to affect the likelihood and extent of teratogenesis are dosage, time of exposure, and genotype of the embryo.

- Fetal alcohol syndrome is perhaps the most common cause of acquired mental retardation.

- Isotretinoin is effective for treatment of cystic acne, but is also considered to be one of the most potent teratogens in widespread use.

## Key Terms

**Amnion:** a membrane that forms a fluid-filled sac around the embryo.

**Blastocyst:** an early stage of embryo development, which can be recognized through the presence of an inner cell mass.

**Ectoderm:** the outer layer of cells in the embryo, after establishment of the three primary germ layers (ectoderm, mesoderm, endoderm); the germ layer that comes in contact with the amniotic cavity.

**Embryo:** the developing human within the first two months after conception.

**Endoderm:** the innermost of the three primary germ layers of the embryo (ectoderm, mesoderm, endoderm). The epithelial lining of the primitive gut tract and the epithelial component of the glands and other structures (e.g., lower respiratory system) that develop as outgrowths from the gut tube are derived from the endoderm.

**Fetal alcohol effect:** the development of relatively mild degrees of mental deficiency and emotional disorders in children whose mothers use alcohol during their pregnancy; this condition is more common than the full fetal alcohol syndrome scenario.

**Hydrocephalus:** a condition marked by an excessive accumulation of cerebrospinal fluid, resulting in dilation of the cerebral ventricles and raised intracranial pressure; it may also result in enlargement of the cranium and atrophy of the brain.

**Inner cell mass (ICM):** the cells at the embryonic pole of the blastocyst, which are concerned with formation of the body of the embryo.

**Mesoderm:** the middle of the three primary germ layers of the embryo (the others being ectoderm and endoderm). The mesoderm is the origin of connective tissues, myoblasts, blood, the cardiovascular and lymphatic systems, most of the urogenital system, and the lining of the pericardial, pleural, and peritoneal cavities.

**Microcephaly:** abnormal smallness of the head; a term applied to a skull with a capacity of less than 1350 mL. Microcephaly is usually associated with mental retardation.

**Morning after pill:** a form of emergency birth control used to prevent a woman from becoming pregnant after she has engaged in unprotected vaginal intercourse.

**Morula:** the earliest stage of embryo after cell division, consisting of a ball of identical cells.

**Organogenesis:** formation of organs during development.

**Paracrines:** a group of chemical messengers that communicate with neighboring cells by simple diffusion.

**Parturition:** the process of birth.

**Phocomelia:** defective development of arms or legs, or both, so that the hands and feet are attached close to the body, resembling the flippers of a seal.

**Placenta:** a structure consisting of maternal and fetal tissues that allows for exchange of gases, nutrients, and wastes between the mother's circulatory system and the circulatory system of the fetus.

**Porencephaly:** the occurrence of cavities in the brain substance, communicating usually with the lateral ventricles.

**Trophoblast:** the cell layer covering the blastocyst that erodes the uterine mucosa and through which the embryo receives nourishment from the mother. The cells do not enter into the formation of the embryo itself, but rather contribute to the formation of the placenta.

**Yolk sac:** the sac of extraembryonic membrane that is located ventral to the embryonic disk and, after formation of the gut tube, is connected to the midgut; by the second month of development, this connection has become the narrow yolk stalk. The yolk sac is the first hematopoietic organ of the embryo.

**Zygote:** fertilized ovum before cleavage begins.

## Chapter Review Questions

1. The _____ attaches to the uterine wall six or seven days after fertilization.

2. After the amnion is formed, the cells of the inner cell mass differentiate to create three distinct germ layers: the _____, the _____, and the _____.

3. The critical period for teratogenic effects is between _____ of gestation.

4. Which drug was given to pregnant women to prevent morning sickness between weeks 4 and 10 and caused severe birth defects?

5. A complex of similar signs and symptoms produced by fetal or neonatal infection with a variety of microorganisms is referred to as TORCH. What does this acronym refer to?

## Resources

AllRefer.com. Rubella Syndrome: Disease and Conditions. Available at http:// health .allrefer.com/health/congenital-rubella-rubella-syndrome.html. Accessed January 27, 2010.

Azaïs-Braesco V, Pacal G. Vitamin A in Pregnancy: Requirements and Safety Limits. *American Journal of Clinical Nutrition.* 71(suppl):1325S–1333S; 2000.

Chabner BA, Amrein PC, Druker BJ, Michaelson MD, Mitsiades CS, Goss PE, et al. Antineoplastic Agents. In: Brunton LL, Lazo JS, Parker KL (Eds.), *Goodman & Gilman's The Pharmacological Basis of Therapeutics,* 11th ed. New York: McGraw-Hill; 2005. http://www.accessmedicine.com/content.aspx?aID=957513.

Chiras DD. *Human Biology,* 5th ed. Sudbury, MA: Jones and Bartlett; 2005.

Crombleholme WR. Obstetrics. In: McPhee SJ, Papadakis MA, Tierney LM Jr. (Eds.), *Current Medical Diagnosis and Treatment,* 46th ed. New York: McGraw-Hill; 2007, pp. 782–806.

Cunningham FG, Leveno KL, Bloom SL, Hauth JC, Gilstrap LC III, Wenstrom KD. Teratology, Drugs, and Other Medications. In: Cunningham FG, Leveno KL, Bloom SL, Hauth JC, Gilstrap LC III, Wenstrom KD (Eds.), *Williams Obstetrics,* 22nd ed. New York: McGraw-Hill; 2006. http://www.accessmedicine.com/ content .aspx?aID=722628.

FamilyDoctor.org. Cytomegalovirus. http://familydoctor.org/online/famdocen/ home/common/infections/common/viral/743.printerview.html.

Franks ME, Macpherson GR, Figg WD. Thalidomide. *Lancet.* 363:1802–811; 2004.

Germann WJ, Stanfield CL. *Principles of Human Physiology,* 2nd ed. San Francisco, CA: Benjamin Cummings; 2005.

IQ Comparison Site. http://www.iqcomparisonsite.com/IQBasics.aspx.

Medline Plus. Cytomegalovirus Infections. http://www.nlm.nih.gov/medlineplus/ cytomegalovirusinfections.html.

Medline Plus. Rubella. http://www.nlm.nih.gov/medlineplus/rubella.html.

Rubin E. *Essential Pathology,* 3rd ed. Baltimore, MD: Lippincott Williams & Wilkins; 2001.

Smithells RW, Newman CG. Recognition of Thalidomide Defects. *Journal of Medical Genetics.* 29:716–723; 1992.

*Stedman's Online Medical Dictionary.* http://www.stedmans.com/.

Thalidomide Victims Association of Canada. Thalidomide. The Canadian Tragedy. Available at http://www.thalidomide.ca/the-canadian-tragedy/. Accessed January 27, 2010.

# Chapter 4

# Neurodegenerative Diseases

## CHAPTER OBJECTIVES

✓ Describe the etiology and various forms of Alzheimer's disease.

✓ Detail symptoms associated with Alzheimer's disease.

✓ Describe the etiology and symptoms of Huntington's disease.

✓ Review current treatment recommendations for both degenerative diseases.

## Alzheimer's Disease

Dementia is a brain disorder that seriously affects the ability of a person to perform daily activities. The most common form of dementia in older people is Alzheimer's disease (AD), which involves progressive mental deterioration manifested by memory loss, ability to calculate, loss of visual–spatial orientation, confusion, and disorientation. The disease usually begins after age 60 and the risk increases with age; AD results in death within 5 to 10 years.

People affected by Alzheimer's disease have a loss of cholinergic neurons in certain brain areas and exhibit the formation of plaques and tangles in these neurons. The brain is also atrophic. Both of these effects are believed to block the normal communication between nerve cells.

Alzheimer's disease accounts for approximately 65% of dementia cases in the United States, with the rest primarily attributable to vascular dementia. Risk factors for AD include greater age, family history, lower education level, and female gender. Some measures that may slow down the progression of the disease include nonsteroidal anti-inflammatory drugs, HMG-CoA reductase inhibitors (statins), moderate ethanol intake, and strong social support. Unfortunately, there is no cure for this devastating disease; it gets worse over time and is inevitably fatal. It has been predicted that AD will become a public health crisis of the twenty-first century as baby boomers grow older. The total number of people with this disease in the United States will explode from an estimated 5.1 million today to as many as 11 million to 16 million by 2050.

## Diagnostic Clues

Progressive impairment of intellectual function, including short-term memory loss and one or more deficits in at least one other area such as aphasia, apraxia, agnosia, or a disturbance in executive functioning, are common clinical features of AD. Alzheimer's disease typically presents with early problems in memory and visuospatial abilities (e.g., becoming lost in familiar surroundings, inability to copy a geometric design on paper). Social graces may be retained despite advanced cognitive decline. Personality changes and behavioral difficulties (e.g., wandering, inappropriate sexual behavior, agitation, and aggressiveness) may develop as the disease progresses. Hallucinations may occur in moderate to severe dementia. It is important to note that delirium is not usually associated with Alzheimer's disease. End-stage disease is characterized by near-mutism; inability to sit up, hold up the head, or track objects with the eyes; difficulty with eating and swallowing; weight loss; bowel or bladder incontinence; and recurrent respiratory or urinary tract infections.

## Genetic Progress

Research has shown that those persons who have a parent, brother or sister, or child with AD are more likely to develop AD. These observations support the involvement of genetics and/or environment as factors influencing the development of AD. In fact, several different genes appear to predispose persons to development of AD when they are mutated.

Two forms of Alzheimer's genes have been identified. In "familial Alzheimer's disease," many family members in multiple generations are affected. This type of AD is also referred to as "early onset" because symptoms start before age 65 and are caused by mutations on chromosomes 1, 14, or 21. All of these genes influence production of beta-amyloid, a sticky protein fragment that clumps together in the brain. Fortunately, mutations in these genes are rare and account for less than 5% of all AD cases. Because all children have a 50% chance of developing early-onset AD if one of their parents had it, the inheritance pattern is autosomal dominant.

The second form of AD is late-onset or sporadic Alzheimer's disease; this variation, which accounts for the majority of cases, usually develops after age 65. Even though a specific gene has not been identified as a specific cause of this form of the disease, one gene appears to influence the risk of developing the disease. The apolipoprotein E (APOE) gene found on chromosome 19 is involved in making a protein that helps carry cholesterol in the bloodstream; this protein may also be involved in determining the structure and function of the fatty membrane surrounding a brain cell.

Although the APOE gene has several different forms (**alleles**), three occur most frequently: APOE e2, APOE e3, and APOE e4. People inherit one APOE allele from each parent. The presence of one or two copies of e4 increases AD risk in an individual. While having this allele is a risk factor, it does not mean that AD will always develop. Some people with two copies of e4 do not develop clinical signs of AD, whereas others with no e4s do. Between 35% and 50% of people with AD have at least one copy of APOE e4. These results suggest that other currently unidentified genes are also involved in the propensity to develop AD, as well as environmental factors.

## Diagnostic Testing

Even though individuals who carry the APOE e4 allele are at increased risk of developing late-onset AD, APOE testing is not recommended because there is no way to tell whether a person with this allele will definitely develop the disease. The only definitive way to diagnose AD is to microscopically examine brain tissue (from a postmortem autopsy) to determine if there are plaques and tangles present. Clinical evaluation should include a family history, medical history, laboratory tests, mini-mental status exam, and neuroimaging. If no other cause for the dementia is identified, a person is said to have "probable" or "possible" AD.

## Treatment

In recognition of the loss of cholinergic neurons associated with this disease (i.e., loss of the neurotransmitter acetylcholine), acetylcholinesterase inhibitors (donepezil, galantamine, rivastigmine) have been used to treat patients with mild to moderate AD. These drugs increase the amount of acetylcholine available in the brain by blocking its destruction by acetylcholinesterase in synaptic spaces. These medications produce modest improvements in cognitive function.

Patients with moderate to severe disease have shown benefit from the use of memantine, which is an *N*-methyl-D-aspartase (NMDA) receptor antagonist. It is believed that too much of the neurotransmitter glutamate in the brain can lead to nerve degeneration and contribute to AD. Memantine blocks the glutamate receptor (NMDA), thereby decreasing the excess stimulatory effect of glutamate. Its use has produced moderate improvement in cognitive function when compared to baseline. In addition, memantine can be combined with use of an acetylcholinesterase inhibitor.

# Huntington's Disease

Huntington's disease (HD; also known as Huntington's chorea) is a progressive neurodegenerative disease that is not reversible. This autosomal dominant disorder is characterized by involuntary movements of all parts of the body, deterioration of cognitive function, and, often, severe emotional disturbance. As in other autosomal dominant disorders, if one parent has HD, each offspring has a 50% chance of developing the disease. Similar to the relationship between AD and plaque, HD involves microscopic deposits of amyloid-related protein in the basal ganglia. The name **chorea** refers to "ceaseless rapid complex body movements that look well coordinated and purposeful but are, in fact, involuntary" (MedicineNet, 2010). The period of time from the onset of symptoms to death averages 15 years.

## Genetics

This disorder primarily affects white people of northwestern European ancestry. The HD gene on chromosome 4 codes for a novel protein termed **Huntingtin**; the mutation in HD consists of an expanded and unstable trinucleotide (CAG) repeat. In most autosomal dominant diseases, heterozygotes tend to be less severely affected than homozygotes. However, HD is an exception and appears to be the only human disorder of complete dominance (**Figure 4-1**). Most cases are inherited, but some new cases occur as spontaneous mutations.

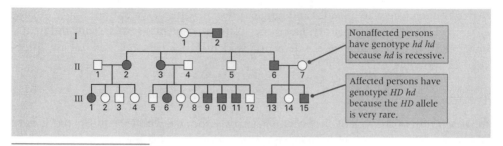

**Figure 4-1** Pedigree of a human family showing the inheritance of the dominant gene for Huntington's disease. Females and males are represented by circles and squares. Shaded symbols indicate people affected with the disease.

The genetic injury remains latent for three to five decades, after which it manifests itself in the form of progressive neuronal dysfunction. The sex of the affected parent exerts a strong influence on the expression of HD. Specifically, inheritance of the HD allele from an affected father results in clinical disease three years earlier than inheritance of the allele from an affected mother. Furthermore, children with juvenile-onset HD have almost always inherited the mutated gene from the father. It is thought that a process that differentially labels maternal and paternal chromosomes (genomic imprinting) plays a role in this early expression.

## Diagnostic Clues

Initial symptoms may consist of either abnormal movements or intellectual changes, but eventually both of these will occur. Onset of symptoms usually occurs between 30 and 50 years of age. The earliest mental changes are often behavioral (i.e., irritability, moodiness, antisocial behavior, or psychiatric disturbance), followed by subsequent dementia. The **dyskinesia** initially may be no more than restlessness, but eventually choreiform movements and dystonic posturing occur. "Progressive rigidity and akinesia (rather than chorea) sometimes occur in association with dementia, particularly in cases of childhood onset" (Aminoff, 2007). **Table 4-1** summarizes the early and late signs and symptoms associated with HD.

## Diagnostic Testing

Clinical evaluation should include a thorough family history and medical history. In established cases of HD, computerized tomography (CT) scanning usually demonstrates cerebral atrophy and atrophy of the caudate nucleus. Magnetic resonance imaging (MRI) and positron emission tomography (PET) have shown reduced glucose utilization in an anatomically normal caudate nucleus. Offspring of known HD-affected parents should be offered genetic counseling. Genetic testing provides for pre-symptomatic detection and definitive diagnosis of the disease.

Table 4-1    **Physical Signs and Symptoms Associated with Huntington's Disease**

| Early | Late |
|-------|------|
| Personality changes | Sudden jerky, involuntary movements throughout body |
| Decreased cognitive abilities | |
| Mild balance problems | Wide, prancing gait |
| Clumsiness | Severe balance and coordination problems |
| Involuntary facial movements | Unable to shift gaze without moving head |
| | Hesitant, halting or slurred speech |
| | Unable to swallow |
| | Dementia |

*Source:* Adapted from Huntington's Disease Symptoms. MayoClinic.com Web site. Available at http://www.mayoclinic.com/health/huntingtons-disease/DS00401/DSECTION=symptoms. Accessed January 16, 2010.

## Treatment

Unfortunately, there is no cure for HD, and disease progression cannot be halted. Treatment is offered purely for symptomatic relief and is aimed at known biochemical changes that suggest under-activity of neurons that contain gamma-aminobutyric acid (GABA) and acetylcholine or a relative over-activity of dopaminergic neurons. Drugs that block dopamine receptors, such as phenothiazines or haloperidol, may control dyskinesia and any behavioral disturbances. However, a common side effect is sedation. In some cases, these medications may cause additional stiffness and rigidity. Attempts to compensate for the relative GABA deficiency by enhancing central GABA activity or to compensate for the relative cholinergic under-activity by giving choline chloride have not been therapeutic.

Because speech can be impaired and affect the ability to express complex thoughts, speech therapy may be beneficial for patients with symptomatic HD. Physical therapy can keep muscles stronger and more flexible, which helps the patient maintain balance and may lessen the risk of falling. Occupational therapy can help make the home safer and provide strategies for coping with memory and concentration problems. Furthermore, later in the course of the disease, occupational therapy can assist with eating, dressing, and hygiene challenges.

## Chapter Summary

- The most common form of dementia in older people is Alzheimer's disease, which involves progressive mental deterioration manifested by memory loss, ability to calculate, loss of visual–spatial orientation, confusion, and disorientation.

- Alzheimer's disease typically presents with early problems in memory and visuo-spatial abilities.

- The majority of Alzheimer's disease cases are late onset or sporadic, usually developing after age 65.

- Acetylcholinesterase inhibitors have been used to treat patients with mild to moderate Alzheimer's disease.

- Huntington's disease is an autosomal dominant disorder characterized by involuntary movements of all parts of the body, deterioration of cognitive function, and, often, severe emotional disturbance.

- There is no cure for Huntington's disease, and disease progression cannot be halted.

## Key Terms

**Allele:** any one of a series of one, two, or more alternative forms of a gene that may occupy the same locus on a specific chromosome.

**Chorea:** from the Greek word for "dance"; the incessant, quick, jerky, involuntary movements that are characteristic of Huntington's disease.

**Dyskinesia:** difficulty in performing voluntary movements.

**Huntingtin:** the product of the Huntington's disease gene on chromosome 4.

## Chapter Review Questions

1. Alzheimer's disease accounts for approximately 65% of dementia cases in the United States, with the rest primarily attributable to _____.

2. Early problems associated with Alzheimer's disease typically include _____ and _____.

3. The majority of Alzheimer's disease is _____, as it usually develops after age 65.

4. The Huntington's disease gene on chromosome 4 codes for a novel protein called _____.

5. The earliest mental changes associated with Huntington's disease are often behavioral followed by subsequent _____.

## Resources

Alzheimer's Association. www.alz.org.

*The Alzheimer's Project.* HBO Documentaries. http://www.hbo.com/alzheimers/index.html.

Aminoff MJ. Nervous System. In: McPhee SJ, Papadakis MA, Tierney LM Jr. *Current Medical Diagnosis and Treatment,* 46th ed. New York: McGraw-Hill; 2007; pp. 998–1062.

Bird TD. Alzheimer Disease Overview. 2008. *GeneReviews.* http:// www.ncbi.nlm.nih .gov/bookshelf/br.fcgi?book=gene&part=alzheimer.

Germann WJ, Stanfield CL. *Principles of Human Physiology,* 2nd ed. New York: Pearson/ Benjamin Cummings; 2005.

Hartl DL, Jones EW. *Essential Genetics: A Genomic Perspective,* 4th ed. Sudbury, MA: Jones and Bartlett; 2006.

Hartl DL, Jones EW. *Genetics: Analysis of Genes and Genomes,* 6th ed. Sudbury, MA: Jones and Bartlett; 2005.

Hughes MD. Multiple Sclerosis, Alzheimer's Disease, and Dementia. *Audio-Digest Family Practice.* 54(16); 2006.

Johnston CB, Covinsky KE, Landefeld CS. Geriatric Medicine. In: Tierney LM, McPhee SJ, Papadakis MA. *Current Medical Diagnosis and Treatment,* 44th ed. New York: McGraw-Hill; 2005.

Mayo Clinic. Huntington's Disease. http://www.mayoclinic.com/health/hunting tons-disease/DS00401. Accessed January 27, 2010.

McConnell TH. The Nature of Disease. In: *Pathology for the Health Professions..* Baltimore, MD: Lippincott Williams & Wilkins; 2007, p. 639.

MedicineNet, Inc. Definition of Chorea. Available at http://www.medterms.com/ script/main/art.asp?articlekey=10029. Accessed January 27, 2010.

MedicineNet.com. Medications and Drugs. http://www.medicinenet.com/meman tine/article.htm. Accessed August 13, 2010.

Rubin E. *Essential Pathology,* 3rd ed. Baltimore, MD: Lippincott Williams & Wilkins; 2001.

*Stedman's Online Medical Dictionary.* http://www.stedmans.com/.

U.S. National Institute of Health National Institute on Aging, Alzheimer's Disease Education and Resource Center. http://www.nia.nih.gov/alzheimers/.

# Chapter 5

# Hereditary Breast and Ovarian Cancer Syndrome

## CHAPTER OBJECTIVES

✓ Describe the genes involved in hereditary breast and ovarian cancer.
✓ Identify risks associated with mutations in breast cancer genes.
✓ Detail the impacts of the founder effect and penetrance.
✓ Discuss management options for patients at risk or affected by
  hereditary breast and/or ovarian cancer.

Cancer accounts for approximately 20% of all deaths in the United States. While genetics certainly plays a role in many different cancers, it is known that most cancer is not inherited. Rather, it is the *predisposition* to cancer that is inherited. Approximately 5% to 10% of breast and ovarian cancers are attributable to known predisposing genetic factors.

The lifetime risk for a woman of developing breast cancer is more than 13% (1 in 7), while the lifetime risk of developing ovarian cancer is a little more than 1% (1 in 58). The lifetime risk for males to develop breast cancer is less than 1%. Epidemiological studies have established the role of family history as an important risk factor for both breast and ovarian cancer. After gender and age, a positive family history is the strongest known predictive risk factor for breast cancer.

Major phenotypic features of hereditary breast and ovarian cancer syndrome include early age (often before age 50) of breast cancer onset, family history of both breast and ovarian cancer, increased chance of bilateral cancers (i.e., both breasts and ovaries), or increased risk of development of both breast and ovarian cancer in the same individual. Other diagnostic clues include an autosomal dominant pattern of inheritance, which means a vertical transmission of cancer through either the maternal or paternal side of the family. An increased incidence of tumors in other specific organs, such as the ovary and prostate, in family members is also consistent with this syndrome. Other factors that increase the likelihood of hereditary breast and ovarian syndrome are a family history of male breast cancer as well as Ashkenazi Jewish ancestry.

## Breast Cancer Genes

The study of large **kindreds** with multiple individuals affected with breast cancer led to the identification of two major cancer susceptibility genes. In 1990, the first gene associated with breast cancer was identified on chromosome 17. This gene was named "breast cancer 1" or **BRCA1**. Mutations in this gene are transmitted through an autosomal dominant pattern in a family. The *BRCA1* gene was found to encode for a protein that contained 1863 amino acids. Even after this significant finding, it was soon apparent that not all families with hereditary breast cancer possessed the *BRCA1* gene. In 1994, another gene (**BRCA2**) was identified on chromosome 13 that encoded a protein consisting of 3418 amino acids. Mutations in this gene are also transmitted in an autosomal dominant familial pattern and are associated with male breast cancer, ovarian cancer, prostate cancer, and pancreatic cancer.

Both *BRCA1* and *BRCA2* are **tumor suppressor genes**, which normally control cell growth and cell death. In addition, both genes are involved in other important cell functions, including DNA repair, genomic stability, transcriptional regulation, and cell cycle control. Each individual has two *BRCA1* genes (one on each chromosome 17) and two *BRCA2* genes (one on each chromosome 13). When a person has one altered or mutated copy of either *BRCA1* or *BRCA2*, his or her risk for various types of cancer increases (**Table 5-1**).

Before cancer will develop in a person, both copies of a tumor suppressor gene (i.e., *BRCA*) must be mutated. For example, in the case of hereditary breast and ovarian cancer syndrome, the first mutation is inherited from either the mother or the father and is present in all body cells. This is called a **germline mutation**. Whether a person with a germline mutation develops cancer and where the cancer appears will depend on where the second mutation occurs. If the second mutation is in the ovary, then ovarian cancer may develop. If it manifests in the breast, then breast cancer may develop.

Even though mutations in tumor suppressor genes are known to increase the risk of developing cancer, tumor development requires mutations in multiple growth control genes to become manifest. Loss of both copies of *BRCA1* or *BRCA2* is just the first step in the overall process of **tumorigenesis**. The causes of these additional mutations are unknown. It has been suggested that chemical, physical, or biological environmental exposures or chance errors in cell replication may be involved.

### Table 5-1  Risks Associated with Either a *BRCA1* or *BRCA2* Mutation

| *BRCA1* Mutation | *BRCA2* Mutation |
| --- | --- |
| Lifetime risk for breast cancer: 36% to 85% | Lifetime risk for breast cancer (females): 36% to 85% |
| Lifetime risk for second breast cancer: 40% to 60% | Lifetime risk for breast cancer (males): 6% |
| Lifetime risk for ovarian cancer: 20% to 60% | Lifetime risk for ovarian cancer: up to 27% |
| Increased risk for other cancer types (i.e., prostate) | Increased risk for other cancer types (i.e., pancreatic, prostate, laryngeal, stomach, and melanoma) |

*Source:* Adapted from Breast Health, Hereditary Breast Ovarian Cancer Syndrome (*BRCA1/BRCA2*). University of Virginia Health System. Available at http://www.healthsystem. virginia.edu/UVAHealth/adult_breast/herbrov.cfm. Accessed September 30, 2009.

Even though an individual may have inherited a germline *BRCA1* or *BRCA2* mutation, that person may never develop cancer because he or she may never get the second mutation that knocks out the function of the gene and starts the process of tumor formation. This phenomenon can make it appear that the cancer has "skipped" a generation within a family, when, in reality, the mutation is present. Regardless of whether they develop cancer, individuals with a mutation have a 50:50 chance of passing the mutation on to the next generation.

Approximately 2000 distinct mutations and sequence variations in *BRCA1* and *BRCA2* have been described. Unfortunately, current mutation screening methods vary in their sensitivity, and no definitive functional tests for *BRCA1* or *BRCA2* are currently available. In addition, 10% to 15% of all individuals undergoing genetic testing with full sequencing of *BRCA1* and *BRCA2* will not have a clearly identifiable deleterious mutation. Therefore, clinical management of these patients must rely on a thorough personal history as well as the family cancer history.

## Founder Effect

Among those affected with *BRCA1* or *BRCA2* mutations, most families express mutations specific to that family. Mutations in such families that recur for generation after generation have been studied in families of Ashkenazi Jewish heritage as well as in families originating from the Netherlands, Iceland, and Sweden. This pattern represents the **founder effect**. Three mutations account for the majority of the *BRCA* mutations in individuals of Ashkenazi Jewish ancestry (**Table 5-2**). These three mutations are thought to occur at an increased rate due to a combination of founder effect and genetic drift. In other words, these mutations are assumed to have originated in a common ancestor shared by many Ashkenazi Jews. Founder effect mutations for *BRCA1* and *BRCA2* are also seen in Dutch, Icelandic, Swedish, and Japanese populations. Based on this information, some laboratories offer "ethnic-specific" mutation genetic testing panels. Such tests look for specific mutations based on the ethnicity of a patient rather than searching through the entire gene sequence.

**Table 5-2  Mutations Associated with Breast and Ovarian Cancer in the Ashkenazi Jewish Population**

| Mutation | Gene | Carrier Frequency in Ashkenazi Jewish Population |
|---|---|---|
| 185delAG | *BRCA1* | 0.9% |
| 5382insC | *BRCA1* | 0.3% |
| 6174delT | *BRCA2* | 1.3% |

*Source:* Data from Major Genes. *Genetics of Breast and Ovarian Cancer (PDQ®).* National Cancer Institute. U.S. National Institutes of Health. Available at http://www.cancer.gov/cancertopics/pdq/genetics/breast-and-ovarian. Accessed January 16, 2010.

In the general population, it has been estimated that 1 in 800 individuals has a *BRCA1* or *BRCA2* mutation. In contrast, due to the founder effect, 1 in 40 Ashkenazi individuals has one of the recurring mutations. Obviously, this knowledge has important implications in terms of assessing family history for breast and ovarian cancer in Ashkenazi versus non-Ashkenazi individuals.

## Penetrance

Penetrance is defined as the probability of developing disease in a carrier of a deleterious mutation; it is usually defined in terms of a given age (e.g., to age 70). To estimate risk, penetrance of certain mutations must be understood. Modifiers are also affected by penetrance.

Thus the relative risk of developing a major disorder is calculated by comparison of the incidence of a condition associated with a specific gene mutation among carriers of that mutation in relationship to the incidence among noncarriers of the mutation. The risk of cancer among individuals who carry a mutation in *BRCA1* or *BRCA2* may be modified by a second gene or by an environmental factor. Examples of these environmental factors include exposure to carcinogens (i.e., tobacco) and hormonal factors. For modifying factors, the relative risk is the penetrance of the disease among individuals with the modifying factor compared to the penetrance of the disease among those without the modifying factor. Estimates of penetrance by age 70 years for *BRCA1* and *BRCA2* cover a large range, from 14% to 87% for breast cancer and from 10% to 68% for ovarian cancer.

## Rare Syndromes Associated with Breast and Ovarian Cancer

**Li-Fraumeni syndrome** is a rare syndrome associated with a germline mutation on chromosome 17. It is characterized by premenopausal breast cancer in combination with childhood sarcoma, brain tumors, leukemia, and adrenocortical carcinoma. Tumors in families who carry the Li-Fraumeni syndrome mutation tend to occur in childhood and early adulthood and often present as multiple primary tumors in the same individual. The average age of onset of breast cancer is 34.6 years in families with this mutation.

**Cowden syndrome** is characterized by multiple hamartomas, an excess of breast cancer, gastrointestinal malignancies, endometrial cancer, and both benign and malignant thyroid disease. Lifetime estimates for breast cancer among woman with this syndrome range between 25% and 50%. Onset is often at a young age and may be bilateral. Skin manifestations include multiple trichilemmomas, oral fibromas and papillomas, and acral, palmar, and plantar keratoses. Germline mutations on chromosome 10 are responsible for this syndrome.

**Peutz-Jeghers syndrome** is characterized by melanocytic macules on the lips, perioral, and buccal regions, along with multiple gastrointestinal polyps. Mutations at chromosome 19 in a tumor suppressor gene have been identified as one cause of this disease. The gastrointestinal tract is commonly affected, with a cumulative incidence of gastrointestinal cancer by age 70. In addition, one study showed that the cumulative risk of breast cancer was 31% by age 60.

## Management Options

### Breast Imaging

Given that there is only limited information detailing outcomes of interventions to reduce risk in patients with a genetic susceptibility to breast or ovarian cancer, recommendations in this area are primarily based on expert opinion. The Cancer Genetics Studies Consortium task force has recommended that female carriers of a *BRCA1* or *BRCA2* high-risk mutation get "annual mammography, beginning at age 25 to 35 years. Mammograms should be done at a consistent location when possible, with prior films available for comparison." Because *BRCA1* and *BRCA2* proteins are known to play a role in repairing DNA damage (including radiation damage), it has been suggested that *BRCA* mutation carriers may be more susceptible to radiation-induced breast cancer compared to women without mutations. However, there is insufficient evidence to suggest that mutation carriers should avoid mammography.

Magnetic resonance imaging (MRI) has also been investigated as a screening tool for breast cancer. Studies consistently demonstrate that breast MRI is more sensitive than either mammography or ultrasound for the detection of hereditary breast cancer. However, mammography has been shown to identify some cancers (ductal carcinomas in situ) that are not identified by MRI. Consequently, the American Cancer Society recommends annual MRI screening in addition to mammography for women at hereditary risk for breast cancer.

### Mastectomy

Several studies have evaluated the effectiveness of risk-reducing mastectomy in women with *BRCA1* or *BRCA2* mutations. In one study, bilateral mastectomy reduced the risk of breast cancer in *BRCA1/BRCA2* mutation carriers after a mean follow-up of 6.4 years by approximately 90%. Whether a woman elects to have risk-reducing mastectomy depends on several factors, including age, culture, geography, healthcare system, insurance coverage, provider attitudes, and other social factors.

### Ovarian Cancer Screening

Current recommendations for women with a higher, inherited risk of ovarian cancer include annual or semiannual screening using transvaginal ultrasound and serum CA-125 levels. This guideline is based on the observation that elevated serum CA-125 levels are associated with ovarian tumors. Unfortunately, neither of these screening techniques has been shown to detect ovarian cancer at an early and potentially more treatable stage. Therefore, prophylactic bilateral salpingo-oophorectomy is recommended between the ages of 35 to 40 years or upon completion of childbearing as an effective (approximately 95%) risk-reduction option.

## Genetic Testing

While genetic tests are available that can identify mutations in *BRCA1/BRCA2*, it is preferable to first test an individual who is affected by cancer before testing unaffected family members. This step is taken to determine whether a detectable *BRCA1* or *BRCA2* mutation is responsible for the breast and/or ovarian cancer within a family. If an unaffected family member is then tested for a known mutation, two results are possible: (1) positive: the individual is at increased risk to develop breast and ovarian cancer; or (2) negative: the individual is not at increased risk but still has the general population risk (approximately 13%). Unfortunately, a negative result may also mean that a mutation is present that was not detected due to limitations of the test, or this individual may have a mutation in a different gene that predisposes the person to breast and/or ovarian cancer. Clearly, in addition to benefits, there are limitations associated with genetic testing (**Table 5-3**).

There are many statistical software programs available for assessing the probability that an individual carries a germline deleterious mutation of the *BRCA1* and *BRCA2* genes. For an example, see http://astor.som.jhmi.edu/BayesMendel/index.html. This statistical model is based on family history of breast and ovarian cancer including male breast cancer. It provides updated penetrance estimates for breast and ovarian cancers, and oophrectomy history can be included in the model as well as molecular marker information. Based on the time limitations associated with each patient encounter, it is unlikely that many primary care practitioners would utilize this type of software. Instead, it is more likely to be used by genetic counselors.

## Chapter Summary

- After gender and age, a positive family history is the strongest known predictive risk factor for breast cancer.

Table 5-3 **Benefits, Risks, and Limitations of *BRCA* Testing**

| Benefits | Limitations |
| --- | --- |
| Identifies high-risk individuals | Does not detect all mutations |
| Identifies noncarriers in families with a known mutation | Continued risk of sporadic cancer |
| Allows early detection and prevention strategies | May result in psychosocial and/or economic harm |
| May relieve anxiety | |

*Source:* Adapted from Armstrong et al. (2000) and BRCA1 and BRCA2: Cancer Risk and Genetic Testing. National Cancer Institute. U.S. National Institutes of Health. Available at http://www.cancer.gov/cancertopics/factsheet/ risk/brca. Accessed January 16, 2010.

- Two breast cancer genes—*BRCA1* and *BRCA2*—have been identified as playing roles in hereditary breast and ovarian cancer syndrome.
- Both *BRCA1* and *BRCA2* are tumor suppressor genes that normally control cell growth and cell death.
- When a small group of people interbreeds over generations, specific rare mutations can recur and become more common within the population.
- Even though an individual may have inherited a germline *BRCA1* or *BRCA2* mutation, the person may never develop cancer because he or she may never get the second mutation that knocks out the function of the gene and starts the process of tumor formation.

## Key Terms

**BRCA1:** a tumor suppressor gene on chromosome 17 that prevents cells with damaged DNA from dividing. Carriers of germline mutations in *BRCA1* are predisposed to develop both breast and ovarian cancer.

**BRCA2:** a tumor suppressor gene on chromosome 13. Carriers of germline mutations in *BRCA2* have an increased risk, similar to that of carriers of *BRCA1* mutations, of developing breast cancer and a moderately increased risk of ovarian cancer. *BRCA2* families also exhibit an increased incidence of male breast, pancreatic, prostate, laryngeal, and ocular cancers.

**Cowden syndrome:** caused by mutations in the PTEN gene (a tumor suppressor gene), this syndrome is associated with noncancerous growths known as hamartomas and malignancies such as breast, thyroid and endometrial cancer.

**Founder effect:** accumulation of random genetic changes in an isolated population as a result of its proliferation from only a few parent colonizers.

**Germline mutation:** a change in a gene in the body's reproductive cell (egg or sperm) that becomes incorporated into the DNA of every cell in the body of the offspring.

**Kindred:** an aggregate of genetically related persons.

**Li-Fraumeni syndrome:** caused by a mutation in the p53 gene (a tumor suppressor gene), this syndrome is associated with an increased risk for breast cancer, osteosarcoma and soft tissue sarcomas as well as leukemias and adrenal carcinoma.

**Peutz-Jeghers syndrome:** caused by a mutationi nt he STK11 gene (a tumor suppressor gene), this syndrome is associated with growths of hamartomas in the stomach and intestine, dark freckling in the axilla, perioral area and buccal mucosa, and an increased risk for developing pancreatic, gastrointestinal, ovarian and breast cancers.

**Tumor suppressor gene:** a gene whose function is to suppress cellular proliferation. Loss of a tumor suppressor gene through chromosomal aberration leads to heightened susceptibility to neoplasia.

**Tumorigenesis:** production of a new growth or growths.

## Chapter Review Questions

1. After gender and age, what is the strongest known predictive risk factor for breast cancer?

2. Vertical transmission of a trait through either the maternal or paternal side of the family is indicative of which type of inheritance?

3. _____ is characterized by melanocytic macules on the lips, perioral, and buccal regions along with multiple gastrointestinal polyps.

4. The American Cancer Society recommends annual _____ screening in addition to mammography for women at hereditary risk for breast cancer.

5. When a small group of people interbreeds over generations, specific rare mutations can recur and become more common within the population. This phenomenon is called _____.

## Resources

Armstrong K, Calzone K, Stopfer J, et al. Factors Associated with Decisions About Clinical *BRCA1/2* Testing. *Cancer Epidemiology, Biomarkers & Prevention.* 9:1251–1254; 2000.

Breast Health. Hereditary Breast and Ovarian Cancer Syndrome (*BRCA1/BRCA2*). http://www.healthsystem.virginia.edu/uvahealth/ adult_breast/herbrov.cfm.

Dictionary.com. http://dictionary.reference.com/.

Narod SA. Modifiers of Risk of Hereditary Breast and Ovarian Cancer. *Nature Reviews.* 2:113–123; 2001.

National Cancer Institute. *Dictionary of Cancer Terms.* http://www.cancer.gov/ dictionary/.

National Cancer Institute. Genetics of Breast and Ovarian Cancer. http://www .cancer .gov/cancertopics/pdq/genetics/breast-and-ovarian.

Overview of Cancer Genetics. http://cancer-risk.bsd.uchicago.edu.

Saslow D, Boetes C, Burke W, et al. American Cancer Society Guidelines for Breast Screening with MRI as an Adjunct to Mammography. *CA: A Cancer Journal for Clinicians.* 57:75–89; 2007.

*Stedman's Online Medical Dictionary.* http://www.stedmans.com/.

Westman JA. *Medical Genetics for the Modern Clinician.* New York: Lippincott Williams & Wilkins; 2006.

# Chapter 6

# Colorectal Cancer

## CHAPTER OBJECTIVES

✓ Describe signs and symptoms associated with colorectal cancer.
✓ Identify colorectal cancer screening tests.
✓ Differentiate between sporadic versus hereditary colorectal cancer.
✓ Detail genetic causes of familial adenomatous polyposis and
  hereditary nonpolyposis colorectal cancer.

Colorectal cancer (also called colon cancer or rectal cancer) refers to any cancer in the colon from the beginning (at the cecum) to the end (at the rectum). Colorectal cancer occurs when cells that line the colon or the rectum become abnormal and grow in an out-of-control manner. **Polyps** are usually benign growths that protrude from a mucous membrane in the colon and rectum. If left untreated, these **adenomatous** polyps may eventually evolve into cancer.

Like many cancers, colon cancer may occur sporadically in a population or in a familial pattern. In addition, numerous cancer syndromes involve cancer of the colon. While the majority of colon cancers are sporadic and occur randomly, it is important to recognize familial or hereditary patterns early in individuals. Based on this knowledge, screening and management guidelines have been developed for both patients and their relatives. The primary goal of these guidelines is to prevent colorectal cancer as well as other complications associated with these diseases.

Many patients with colorectal cancer do not experience any symptoms until the disease is quite advanced. For this reason, it is important to take a good family history as well as to assess risk factors for all patients. The risk of colon cancer in a **first-degree relative** of an affected individual can increase an individual's lifetime risk of colon cancer anywhere from 2-fold to 4.3-fold. Signs and symptoms of colorectal cancer are listed in **Table 6-1**. Beginning at age 50, both men and women at average risk for developing colorectal cancer should take the American Cancer Society screening tests identified in **Table 6-2**.

## Table 6-1  Signs and Symptoms Associated with Colorectal Cancer

Blood in the stool

Weight loss with no known reason

Diarrhea that is not the result of diet or illness

A long period of constipation

Crampy abdominal pain

*Continues*

61

**Table 6-1 Signs and Symptoms Associated with Colorectal Cancer** *(Continued)*

Change in bowel habits

Persistent decrease in the size or caliber of stool

Frequent feeling of distention in the abdomen or bowel region (gas pain, bloating, fullness, with or without cramping)

Vomiting and continual lack of energy

*Sources:* American Cancer Society. *Detailed Guide: Colon and Rectum Cancer: How Is Colorectal Cancer Diagnosed?* May 2009. http://www.cancer.org/docroot/CRI/content/CRI_2_4_3X_ How_is_colon_and_rectum_cancer_diagnosed.asp?sitearea=; Mayo Clinic Staff. *Colon Polyps: Symptoms.* July 2009. http://www.mayoclinic.com/health/colon-polyps/DS00511/DSECTION =symptoms; *Johns Hopkins Medicine. Familial Adenomatous Polyposis: Introduction.* 2009. http://www .hopkins-gi.org/GDL_Disease.aspx?CurrentUDV=31&GDL_Disease_ID=FA5AAA54-14DE-4A 8E-B535-6191153083E3&GDL_DC_ID=D03119D7-57A3-4890-A717-CF1E7426C8BA.

**Table 6-2 American Cancer Society Screening Tests**

| Tests That Find Polyps and Cancer | Tests That Mainly Find Cancer |
| --- | --- |
| Flexible sigmoidoscopy every 5 years* | Fecal occult blood test (FOBT) every year*† |
| Colonoscopy every 10 years | Fecal immunochemical test (FIT) every year*† |
| Double-contrast barium enema every 5 years* | Stool DNA test (sDNA), interval uncertain* |
| Computerized tomography (CT) colonography (virtual colonoscopy) every 5 years* | |

*Colonoscopy should be done if test results are positive.
†For FOBT or FIT used as a screening test, the take-home multiple sample method should be used. A FOBT or FIT done during a digital rectal exam is not adequate for screening.
*Source:* American Cancer Society. *Colon Cancer: Signs, Symptoms, and Screening.* 2009. http://www.cancer.org/docroot/SPC/content/SPC_1_Colon_Cancer_Signs_Symptoms_and_ Screening.asp.

# Familial Colorectal Cancer

The occurrence of colorectal cancer in more than one family member may be due to chance alone, or it may result from shared exposure to a cancer-causing substance (carcinogen) in the environment or from similar diet or lifestyle factors. It could also mean the potential for developing colorectal cancer has been passed from one generation to the next, although the exact gene involved has not been identified. Relatives of a person with colorectal cancer may be more likely to develop it themselves. It has been estimated that 15% to 30% of colorectal cancers are familial. Familial colon cancer may be a result of single-gene mutations, multiple-gene mutations, or the combined effect of gene mutations and environmental risk factors. A family history of one or more members with frank colorectal cancer or premalignant polyps should be considered significant.

# Hereditary Colorectal Cancer

The hereditary causes of two hereditary colorectal cancer syndromes, **familial adenomatous polyposis (FAP)** and **hereditary nonpolyposis colorectal cancer (HNPCC)**, have been identified. Like other diseases, colon cancer may occur sporadically, in familial patterns, or such that kindreds have the exact same mutations among those persons affected in a family. Mutations in cancer susceptibility genes predispose a person to inherited types of colorectal cancers. Patterns within a family that exist without the identification of a specific mutation are considered familial colorectal cancers.

# Familial Adenomatous Polyposis

Gardener's syndrome is a phenotypic variant of FAP that manifests as bumps or lumps on the bones of the legs, arms, skull, and jaw; cysts of the skin; teeth that do not erupt when they should; and freckle-like spots on the inside lining of the eyes.

The majority of people with FAP have inherited it. In the other patients affected by this disease, it may be the first case in the family (sporadic). Attenuated FAP is a variant form of FAP in which affected individuals develop fewer polyps (0 to 500), typically at a later age, than those persons with classical FAP. Although people with attenuated FAP tend to develop colon cancer at a later age than individuals with classical FAP, they still have a near 100% lifetime risk of colon cancer.

People with FAP have a 50% chance of passing the condition to each of their children. The condition can be passed on to offspring even if the patient has had his or her own colon removed. In contrast, children who do not inherit the condition from their parent cannot pass it to their own children. Approximately one third of people with FAP do not have an affected parent. Individuals who inherit a mutated **adenomatous polyposis coli** (*APC*) gene have a very high likelihood of developing colonic **adenomas**; this risk has been estimated to be more than 90%. The age of onset of adenomas is variable. By age 10 years, only 15% of FAP gene carriers manifest adenomas; by age 20 years, the probability rises to 75%; and by age 30 years, 90% will have presented with FAP.

## Genetics of Familial Adenomatous Polyposis

Familial adenomatous polyposis is an autosomal dominant condition caused by mutations in the *APC* tumor suppressor gene on chromosome 5. Most of these mutations lead to premature stop codons that result in truncation of the *APC* gene product, a protein that plays an important role in the regulation of cell adhesion and **apoptosis**. More than 800 different mutations have been reported. The majority of these changes are **insertions**, **deletions**, and **nonsense mutations** that lead to **frameshift** and/or premature stop codons during gene transcription. The location of the mutation affects the number of polyps formed and the type of extracolonic features seen.

Recently, mutations in the *MYH* gene—a gene involved with base excision repair—have been identified in patients with the classic and attenuated forms of FAP who do not have mutations of the *APC* gene. The FAP caused by *MYH* mutation is inherited in an autosomal recessive fashion; hence a family history of colorectal cancer may not be evident. Of patients with classic FAP, approximately 90% have a mutation in the *APC* gene and 8% in the *MYH* gene. In contrast, among patients with 10 to 100 adenomatous polyps and suspected attenuated FAP, *APC* mutations are identified in 15% but *MYH* mutations in 25%.

## Genetic Counseling and Testing

Genetic counseling and testing should be offered to patients with a diagnosis of FAP that has been established by endoscopy and to all at-risk relatives of patients with the disease. Testing should also be done to confirm a diagnosis of attenuated disease in patients with 20 or more adenomas. Commercial *APC* gene testing is available. Genetic testing is best performed by sequencing the *APC* gene to identify disease-associated mutations, which are found in approximately 90% of cases of typical FAP. Mutational assessment of *MYH* should be considered in patients with negative test results and in patients with suspected attenuated FAP. Children of patients with FAP should undergo genetic screening beginning at age 10 years.

## Screening Recommendations

If genetic testing cannot be done or is not informative, family members at risk should undergo yearly colonoscopy beginning at 12 years of age. Once the diagnosis has been established, complete **proctocolectomy** or **colectomy** is recommended, usually before age 20 years. Sulindac and cyclooxygenase-2 selective agents have been shown to decrease the number and size of polyps in the rectum but not in the duodenum. Upper endoscopic evaluation of the stomach, duodenum, and peri-ampullary area should be performed every 1 to 3 years to look for adenomas or carcinoma.

If attenuated FAP is suspected within a family, it is important that family members be screened with colonoscopy rather than flexible sigmoidoscopy because polyps are not evenly distributed throughout the colon. Given that the number of polyps and age of onset can vary greatly from one family member to another in a family with attenuated FAP, screening should begin at age 15 and be repeated every 1 to 3 years.

# Hereditary Nonpolyposis Colorectal Cancer

Hereditary nonpolyposis colorectal cancer is also known as Lynch syndrome. "Nonpolyposis" means that colorectal cancer can occur when only a small number of polyps are present or when none at all are present. In families with HNPCC, cancer usually affects the right side of the colon. It often occurs at a younger age than colon cancer that is not inherited. Other cancers may arise in these families as well, including cancer of the uterus, ovaries, stomach, urinary tract, small bowel, and bile ducts.

This autosomal dominant condition accounts for 3% to 5% of all colorectal cancers. Affected individuals have a 60% to 80% lifetime risk of developing colorectal carcinoma and a more than 40% lifetime risk of developing endometrial cancer. Unlike individuals with FAP, patients with HNPCC develop only a few adenomas. In contrast to the traditional polyp → cancer progression (which may take more than 10 years), the polyps in HNPCC are believed to undergo rapid transformation from normal tissue → adenoma → cancer.

Research criteria used to define Lynch syndrome were originally developed in 1990 and referred to as the **Amsterdam criteria**; these criteria were revised in 1999 and are now called the Amsterdam criteria II. The latter criteria include the following specifications to warrant a diagnosis of HNPCC:

1. There should be at least three relatives with a Lynch syndrome–associated cancer (colorectal cancer or cancer of the endometrium, small bowel, ureter, or renal pelvis).

2. One should be a first-degree relative of the other two.

3. At least two successive generations should be affected.

4. At least one family member should be diagnosed before age 50 years.

5. Familial adenomatous polyposis should be excluded in the colorectal cancer cases.

6. Tumors should be verified by pathological examination.

## Genetics of Hereditary Nonpolyposis Colorectal Cancer

A defect in one of several genes (*MLH1, MSH2, MSH6,* and *PMS2*) that are important in the detection and repair of DNA base-pair mismatches causes HNPCC. Germline mutations in *MLH1, MSH2,* and *MSH6* account for more than 90% of the known mutations in families with HNPCC. Mutations in any of these mismatch repair genes result in a characteristic phenotypic DNA abnormality known as **microsatellite instability**. In more than 95% of cancers in patients with HNPCC, microsatellite instability is readily demonstrated by expansion or contraction of DNA microsatellites (short, repeated DNA sequences). Microsatellite instability also occurs in 15% of sporadic colorectal cancers, usually due to aberrant methylation of the *MLH1* promoter, which results in decreased gene expression.

## Genetic Counseling and Testing

A thorough family cancer history is essential to identify families whose members may be affected with HNPCC so that appropriate genetic and colonoscopic screening can be offered. Families with suspected HNPCC should be evaluated first by a genetic counselor and should give informed consent in writing before genetic testing is performed. Patients whose families meet any of the revised Bethesda criteria have an increased likelihood of harboring a germline mutation in one of the mismatch repair genes and should be considered for genetic testing. The Bethesda criteria include the following specifications to warrant a diagnosis of HNPCC:

1. Colorectal cancer prior to age 50

2. Synchronous or metachronous colorectal or HNPCC-associated tumor regardless of age (endometrial, stomach, ovary, pancreas, ureter and renal pelvis, biliary tract, brain)

3. Colorectal cancer, plus one or more first-degree relatives with colorectal or HNPCC-related cancer, with one of the cancers occurring prior to age 50

4. Colorectal cancer, plus two or more second-degree relatives with colorectal or HNPCC cancer, regardless of age

5. Tumors with infiltrating lymphocytes, mucinous/signet ring differentiation, or medullary growth pattern in patients younger than 60 years

These criteria will identify more than 90% of mutation-positive HNPCC families.

Tumor tissues of affected individuals or family members meeting the revised Bethesda criteria should undergo immunohistochemical staining for *MLH1, MSH2, MSH6,* and *PMS2* (using commercially available assays) or testing for microsatellite instability (PCR amplification of a panel of DNA markers), or both. Individuals whose tumors have normal immunohistochemical staining or do not have microsatellite instability are unlikely to have germline mutations in mismatch repair genes and do not require further genetic testing. However, if patients have early-age-onset colon cancer or features of hereditary colon cancer syndrome, they should be treated and managed based on their family history; these steps might include intensive cancer surveillance.

Germline testing for gene mutations is positive in greater than 90% of individuals whose tumors show no histochemical staining of one of the mismatch repair genes and in 50% of those patients whose tumors have a high level of microsatellite instability. Germline testing is also warranted in families with a strong history consistent with HNPCC when tumors from affected members are unavailable for assessment. If a mutation is detected in one of the known mismatch genes in a patient with cancer, genetic testing of other at-risk family members is indicated.

## Screening Recommendations

If genetic testing documents an HNPCC gene mutation, affected relatives should be screened with colonoscopy every 1 to 2 years beginning at age 25 (or at an age 5 years younger than the age at diagnosis of the youngest affected family member). If cancer is found, subtotal colectomy followed by annual surveillance of the rectal stump should be performed. Upper endoscopy should be performed every 2 to 3 years to screen for gastric cancer. Women should undergo screening for endometrial and ovarian cancer beginning at age 25 to 35 years with pelvic examination, CA-125 assay, endometrial aspiration, and transvaginal ultrasound. Prophylactic hysterectomy and oophorectomy may be considered, especially in women who have completed their families (i.e., who are done with childbearing). Similarly, consideration should be given for increased cancer surveillance in family members in proven or suspected HNPCC families who do not wish to undergo germline testing.

# Chapter Summary

- Colorectal cancer occurs when cells that line the colon or the rectum become abnormal and grow in an out-of-control manner.

- The risk of colon cancer in a first-degree relative of an affected individual can increase an individual's lifetime risk of colon cancer anywhere from 2-fold to 4.3-fold.

- The genetic causes of two hereditary colorectal cancer syndromes—familial adenomatous polyposis and hereditary nonpolyposis colorectal cancer—have been identified.

- If attenuated familial adenomatous polyposis is suspected within a family, it is important that family members be screened with colonoscopy rather than flexible sigmoidoscopy because polyps are not evenly distributed throughout the colon.

## Key Terms

**Adenoma:** a benign epithelial neoplasm in which the tumor cells form glands or gland-like structures.

**Adenomatous:** relating to an adenoma, and to some types of glandular hyperplasia.

**Adenomatous polyposis coli (APC):** a tumor suppressor gene on chromosome 5. Mutations in this gene result in familial adenomatous polyposis.

**Amsterdam criteria:** research criteria for defining Lynch syndrome established by the International Collaborative Group meeting in Amsterdam.

**Apoptosis:** programmed or gene-directed cell death.

**Colectomy:** surgical excision of part or all of the colon.

**Deletion:** absence of a segment of DNA; it may be as small as a single base or large enough to encompass one or more entire genes.

**Familial adenomatous polyposis (FAP):** an inherited colorectal cancer syndrome that leads to hundreds—sometimes even thousands—of polyps in the colon and rectum at a young age.

**First-degree relative:** any relative who is one meiosis away from a particular individual in a family (i.e., parent, sibling, offspring).

**Frameshift mutation:** an insertion or deletion involving a number of base pairs that is not a multiple of three and consequently disrupts the triplet reading frame, usually leading to the creation of a premature termination (stop) codon and resulting in a truncated protein product.

**Hereditary nonpolyposis colorectal cancer (HNPCC):** an inherited colorectal cancer syndrome in which only a small number of polyps are present or not present at all. Also known as Lynch syndrome.

**Insertion:** a chromosome abnormality in which material from one chromosome is inserted into another nonhomologous chromosome; a mutation in which a segment of DNA is inserted into a gene or other segment of DNA, potentially disrupting the coding sequence.

**Microsatellite instability:** a change that occurs in the DNA of certain cells (e.g., tumor cells) in which the number of repeats of microsatellites (short, repeated sequences of DNA) is different than the number of repeats that appeared in the DNA when it was inherited. The cause of microsatellite instability may be a defect in the ability to repair mistakes made when DNA is copied in the cell.

**Nonsense mutation:** a single base-pair substitution that prematurely codes for a stop in amino acid translation (stop codon).

**Polyp:** a usually nonmalignant growth or tumor protruding from the mucous lining of an organ such as the nose, bladder, or intestine, often causing obstruction.

**Proctocolectomy:** a surgical procedure involving the excision of the colon and rectum and the formation of an ileoanal reservoir or pouch.

## Chapter Review Questions

1. _____ are usually benign growths that protrude from a mucous membrane in the colon and rectum.

2. Gardner's syndrome is a phenotypic variant of _____.

3. When discussing sporadic versus hereditary colorectal cancer, it is important to know that _____ is more common.

4. Hereditary nonpolyposis colorectal cancer is also known as _____.

5. If genetic testing documents a gene mutation associated with hereditary nonpolyposis colorectal cancer, affected relatives should be screened with colonoscopy every _____ years beginning at age 25.

## Resources

Aarnio M, Mecklin J-P, Aaltonen LA, Nyström-Lahti M, Järvinen HJ. Life-time Risk of Different Cancers in Hereditary Non-polyposis Colorectal Cancer (HNPCC) Syndrome. *International Journal of Cancer*. 64:430–433; 1995.

American Cancer Society. http://www.cancer.org/docroot/CRI/CRI_2_1x.asp? rnav =criov&dt=10.

Colon Polyps. MayoClinic.com. http://www.mayoclinic.com/health/colon-polyps/ DS00511/DSECTION=risk-factors.

Dictionary.com. http://dictionary.reference.com/.

*Genetics Home Reference.* http://ghr.nlm.nih.gov/.

Johns Hopkins Gastroenterology and Hepatology Resource Center. http://hopkins-gi.nts.jhu.edu/.

Levin B, Lieberman DA, McFarland B, Smith RA, Brooks D, Andrews KS, et al. Screening and Surveillance for the Early Detection of Colorectal Cancer and Adenomatous Polyps, 2008: A Joint Guideline from the American Cancer Society, the U.S. Multi-Society Task Force on Colorectal Cancer, and the American College of Radiology. *CA: A Cancer Journal for Clinicians*. 58:130–160; 2008.

McQuaid KR. Alimentary Tract. In: McPhee SJ, Papadakis MA, Tierney LM Jr., *Current Medical Diagnosis and Treatment,* 46th ed. New York: McGraw-Hill; 2007, pp. 648–658.

National Cancer Institute. Colon and Rectal Cancer. http://www.cancer.gov/cancertopics/types/colon-and-rectal.

Pagon RA. Genetic Testing: When to Test, When to Refer. American *Family Physician.* 72:33; 2005. http://www.aafp.org/afp/20050701/editorials.html.

*Stedman's Online Medical Dictionary.* http://www.stedmans.com/.

# Chapter 7

# Chronic Myelogenous Leukemia

## CHAPTER OBJECTIVES

✓ Describe hematology associated with chronic myelogenous leukemia.
✓ Detail signs and symptoms associated with chronic myelogenous leukemia.
✓ Define the Philadelphia chromosome.
✓ Provide an overview of current treatments and factors associated with recovery from chronic myelogenous leukemia.

*Leukemia* is the term used to describe a cancer in blood cells that are produced in the bone marrow. Specifically, leukemia of the granulocytic cell line in the bone marrow may be either acute or chronic. **Chronic myelogenous leukemia (CML)** is categorized as a myeloproliferative disorder that is insidious in onset and progresses slowly over many months to years.

Under normal circumstances, the granulocytic cell line is derived from a single pluripotent stem cell. This single stem cell differentiates into red blood cells, platelets, or **granulocytes**. In CML, the abnormal cell line is increased in number, but the cells produced are functionally inert. The greater the tumor burden of these abnormal cells, the less marrow space and resources exist for other cells such as healthy white blood cells, red blood cells, and platelets. This situation results in infections, anemias, and bleeding. Other myeloproliferative disorders include **polycythemia vera**, **myelofibrosis**, and essential **thrombocythemia**.

Early in the course of CML, the patient may be asymptomatic. However, as the disease progresses, it can accelerate into a blast crisis similar to an acute leukemia. In this stage, the patient will present extremely ill with multiple infections, anemia, and bleeding directly proportional to the tumor burden.

## Major Phenotypic Features

The overall incidence of CML in the United States is 1.5 cases per 100,000 population, which represents approximately 4000 cases annually. CML occurs more frequently in men than in women. The median age at presentation is 55 years, so CML is regarded as a disorder associated with middle age.

Fatigue, night sweats, and fever are typically the chief complaints of patients presenting with CML (**Table 7-1**). At other times, patients complain of abdominal fullness related to splenomegaly. It is also possible for patients to not have any symptoms. In some cases, an elevated white blood count (usually greater than 25,000/$\mu$L) is discovered incidentally,

**Table 7-1 Signs and Symptoms Associated with Chronic Myelogenous Leukemia**

Feeling very tired

Unexplained weight loss

Fever

Night sweats

Pain or a feeling of fullness below the ribs on the left side

*Source:* Adapted from General Information About Chronic Myelogenous Leukemia. Chronic Myelogenous Leukemia Treatment (PDQ®). National Cancer Institute. U.S. National Institutes of Health.
Available at http://www.cancer.gov/cancertopics/pdq/treatment/CML. Accessed January 16, 2010.

with the increase due to greater presence of granulocytes and their precursors (i.e., bands
and mature forms). On examination, the spleen is enlarged (often markedly so), and
sternal tenderness may be a sign of marrow overexpansion. In cases discovered during
routine laboratory monitoring, these findings are often absent.

## Genetics of Chronic Myelogenous Leukemia

Chronic myelogenous leukemia is characterized by a chromosomal abnormality referred
to as the **Philadelphia chromosome**, which involves a reciprocal translocation between
the long arms of chromosomes 9 and 22. A large portion of chromosome 22 is translocated to chromosome 9, and a smaller piece of chromosome 9 is moved to chromosome
22. The portion of chromosome 9 that is translocated contains the **proto-oncogene** *abl*.
The *abl* gene is received at a specific site on chromosome 22 referred to as the break point
cluster (bcr). The resulting fusion gene *bcr/abl* produces a novel protein that differs from
the normal transcript of the *abl* gene in that it possesses tyrosine kinase activity. This
enzyme causes too many stem cells to develop into white blood cells (granulocytes or
blasts). It is unknown what induces the translocation represented by the Philadelphia
chromosome. No clear correlation with exposure to cytotoxic drugs has been found, and
no evidence suggests a viral etiology for this mutation.

The Philadelphia chromosome is detectable in 90% to 95% of patients with the clinical
and laboratory features of CML. Among the remaining 5% to 10%, the molecular
rearrangement characteristic of CML (*bcr/abl*) can be identified in 30% to 50% by molecular detection methods. The remaining cases comprise a heterogeneous group of disorders of unknown biology and with poor prognosis. Evidence that the *bcr/abl* fusion gene
is pathogenic is provided by transgenic mouse models in which introduction of the gene
almost invariably lead to leukemia.

Cytogenetic analysis (karyotype) is needed in all cases at diagnosis. This type of testing
requires bone marrow aspiration, which will identify not only the presence of the Philadelphia chromosome but also the existence of other chromosomal abnormalities. The
Philadelphia chromosome is usually more readily apparent in marrow metaphases than
in peripheral blood metaphases.

**Fluorescence in situ hybridization (FISH)** may also identify the presence of the *bcr/abl* rearrangement, even if the Philadelphia chromosome cannot be identified by cytogenetic analysis. Another advantage of FISH is that it can be performed with peripheral blood. However, it does not provide information on other chromosomes.

Quantitative polymerase chain reaction (PCR) can also be done at diagnosis to have a baseline measure of the *bcr/abl* transcript levels prior to the start of therapy.

## Phases of Chronic Myelogenous Leukemia

The phase of the disease is assigned based on two factors: (1) the number of immature cells in the blood and bone marrow biopsy and (2) the severity of the patient's symptoms. In the earliest stages, the patient typically has less than 10% blasts in both blood and bone marrow samples. This phase lasts between 2 to 4 years. Once the patient transitions into the accelerated phase, 10% to 20% of the cells in the blood and bone marrow are typically noted to be **blast cells**. Platelet counts decline in this stage and other cytogenetic abnormalities appear. In the final or blastic phase of CML, 20% or more of the cells in the blood or bone marrow are blast cells; this occurs usually within 6 to 8 months. **Blast crisis** describes the cellular criteria of blast phase accompanied by fatigue, fever and splenomegaly. Blast crisis closely resembles acute leukemia, and the median survival at this point is often less than 4 months.

## Treatment

Imatinib mesylate (marketed under the trade name Gleevec) is a good example of targeted molecular therapy for cancer. This drug inhibits the activity of the defective gene in CML: the *bcr/abl* **oncogene**. This activity against the oncogene keeps the number of blast cells low by inducing apoptosis (cell death) in cells with the abnormal oncogene. As a result, it is possible to ameliorate the disease progression of CML in the early phases. Imatinib mesylate also has few side effects and has shown a high response rate in most patients. Favorable response to imatinib mesylate is assessed based on two aspects: (1) regression of blood counts and splenomegaly and (2) cytogenetic testing that reveals diminished activity of the Philadelphia chromosome (**Table 7-2**). The *bcr/abl* gene is measured by PCR assays.

The current goal of therapy for CML is to achieve a good molecular response, with at least a 3-log reduction in the *bcr/abl* level. Patients who achieve this level of molecular response have an excellent prognosis, with 100% of such patients remaining free of disease progression at 6 years. Furthermore, in this favorable-response group, the depth of molecular remission appears to increase over time, leading to the hope that imatinib mesylate might can actually be a curative treatment. Patients with suboptimal molecular responses are best treated by switching from imatinib mesylate to an alternative tyrosine kinase inhibitor such as dasatinib. Dasatinib appears to be a more potent agent and can overcome approximately 90% of the mutations that can form in *bcr/abl* and limit the effectiveness of imatinib mesylate therapy.

Table 7-2  **Response Criteria in Chronic Myelogenous Leukemia**

| Diagnostic Method | Response | Criteria |
|---|---|---|
| Hematologic | Complete | White blood cell count < 10,000 μL, normal morphology; normal hemoglobin and platelet counts |
| | Incomplete | White blood cell count ≥ 10,000 μL |
| Cytogenetic | | Percentage of bone marrow metaphases with Philadelphia chromosome |
| | Complete | 0 |
| | Partial | ≤ 35 |
| | Minor | 36–85 |
| | None | 85–100 |
| Molecular | | Presence of *bcr/abl* transcript |
| | Complete | None |
| | Incomplete | Any |

*Source:* Reproduced from Fauci AS, et al. *Harrison's Manual of Internal Medicine.* 2008.

The only proven curative therapy for CML is allogeneic bone marrow transplantation, which involves a donor and a recipient who are not immunologically identical. However, this approach is not without significant risk. Following allogeneic transplantation, immune cells transplanted with the stem cells or developing from them can react against the patient, causing graft-versus-host disease. Alternatively, if the immunosuppressive preparative regimen used to treat the patient before transplant is inadequate, immuno-competent cells of the patient may lead to graft rejection. The risks of these complications are greatly influenced by the degree of matching between donor and recipient for antigens encoded by genes of the major histocompatibility complex.

The best results (80% cure rate) are obtained in patients who are younger than 40 years of age and transplanted within 1 year after diagnosis from **human leukocyte antigen (HLA)**–matched siblings. Allogeneic transplantation is reserved for patients in whom disease is not well controlled, in whom disease progresses after initial control, or for those who have accelerated phase disease. Time will tell whether the curative potential from transplantation in patients who are initially treated with imatinib mesylate will be com-promised compared to those patients who receive transplantation as initial therapy.

Chemotherapeutic agents can also be used as a treatment option. Hydroxyurea is a ribonucleotide reductase inhibitor that induces rapid disease control. Initial management of patients with chemotherapy is currently reserved for rapid lowering of white blood cells to avoid cerebrovascular events or death from leukostasis, reduction of symptoms, and reversal of symptomatic splenomegaly.

Relapsed CML is characterized by any evidence of progression of disease from a stable remission. Signs of progression may include any of the following: (1) increasing myeloid or blast cells in the peripheral blood or bone marrow, (2) cytogenetic positivity when previously cytogenetic negative, and (3) FISH positivity for *bcr/abl* translocation when previously FISH negative.

Blast crisis CML portends a poor prognosis because the treatments that are effective in chronic-phase CML are generally ineffective in the more severe, acute phase of disease.

## Prognosis

Prior to the introduction of imatinib mesylate therapy in 2001, death was expected in 10% of patients with CML within 2 years and in approximately 20% yearly thereafter; the median survival time was approximately 4 years. Today, more than 80% of patients remain alive and without disease progression at 6 years with the use of imatinib mesylate and other molecular targeted agents. While allogeneic stem cell transplantation is the only proven curative option for CML, some patients may be cured by oral agents. Factors affecting the patient's chance of recovery include patient age, phase of CML, amount of blasts seen in the blood or bone marrow, size of the spleen at diagnosis, and general health of the patient.

## Chapter Summary

- Leukemia is a cancer that starts in blood-forming tissue such as the bone marrow and causes large numbers of blood cells to be produced and enter the bloodstream.
- In chronic myelogenous leukemia, too many blood stem cells develop into abnormal granulocytes.
- A chromosomal abnormality referred to as the Philadelphia chromosome, which involves a reciprocal translocation between the long arms of chromosomes 9 and 22, is associated with chronic myelogenous leukemia.
- The only proven curative therapy for chronic myelogenous leukemia is allogeneic bone marrow transplantation, which involves a donor and a recipient who are not immunologically identical.

## Key Terms

**Blast cells:** an immature precursor cell (e.g., erythroblast, lymphoblast, neuroblast).

**Blast crisis:** in a leukemic patient, a disease stage characterized by fever, fatigue, and clinically poor response to interventions.

**Chronic myelogenous leukemia (CML):** a myeloproliferative disorder characterized by increased proliferation of the granulocytic cell line without the loss of their capacity to differentiate.

**Fluorescence in situ hybridization (FISH):** a analytic technique in which a nucleic acid labeled with a fluorescent dye is hybridized to suitably prepared cells or histological sections; it is then used to look for specific transcription or localization of genes to specific chromosomes.

**Granulocyte:** a mature granular leukocyte, including any of the neutrophilic, acidophilic, and basophilic types of polymorphonuclear leukocytes (i.e., neutrophils, eosinophils, and basophils).

**Human leukocyte antigen (HLA):** system designation for the gene products of at least four linked loci (A, B, C, and D) and a number of subloci on the sixth human chromosome that have been shown to have a strong influence on human allotransplantation, transfusions in refractory patients, and certain disease associations. More than 50 alleles are recognized, most of which are found at loci HLA-A and HLA-B; they are passed on through autosomal dominant inheritance.

**Myelofibrosis:** fibrosis of the bone marrow associated with myeloid metaplasia of the spleen and other organs.

**Oncogene:** any of a family of genes that under normal circumstances code for proteins involved in cell growth or regulation (e.g., protein kinases), but that may foster malignant processes if mutated or activated by contact with retroviruses.

**Philadelphia chromosome:** an abnormal chromosome formed by a rearrangement of chromosomes 9 and 22 that is associated with chronic myelogenous leukemia.

**Polycythemia vera:** a chronic form of polycythemia of unknown cause characterized by bone marrow hyperplasia, an increase in both blood volume and the number of red cells, redness or cyanosis of the skin, and splenomegaly.

**Proto-oncogene:** a gene in the normal human genome that appears to have a role in normal cellular physiology and is involved in regulation of normal cell growth or proliferation; as a result of somatic mutations, these genes may become oncogenic.

**Thrombocythemia:** a primary form of thrombocytopenia, in contrast to secondary forms that are associated with metastatic neoplasms, tuberculosis, and leukemia involving the bone marrow, or occurring as the result of direct suppression of bone marrow by the use of chemical agents.

## Chapter Review Questions

1. The peripheral blood cell profile in patients affected by chronic myelogenous leukemia shows an increased number of _____ and their immature precursors.

2. Patients with CML usually present with fatigue, night sweats, and low-grade fever related to the _____ caused by overproduction of white blood cells.

3. The fusion gene _____ produces a novel protein that differs from the normal gene transcript in that it possesses tyrosine kinase activity.

4. When tiredness, fever, and an enlarged spleen occur during the blastic phase of CML, this situation is called _____ and represents acute leukemia.

5. _____ specifically inhibits the tyrosine kinase activity of the *bcr/abl* oncogene.

# Resources

Fauci AS, Braunwald E, Kasper DL, Hauser SL, Longo DL, Jameson JL, Loscalzo J. *Harrison's Manual of Internal Medicine,* 17th ed. New York: McGraw-Hill Medical; 2008.

Ghelani D, Sneed TB, Bueso-Ramos CE Cortes, J. Chronic Myeloid Leukemia. In: Kantarjian HM, Wolff RA, Koller CA (Eds.), *M. D. Anderson Manual of Medical Oncology.* New York: McGraw-Hill; 2006. http://www.accessmedicine.com/resourceTOC.aspx?resourceID =500.

Lichtman MA, Liesveld JL. Chronic Myelogenous Leukemia and Related Disorders. In: Lichtman MA, Beutler E, Kipps TJ, Seligsohn U, Kaushansky K, Prchal JR. *Williams Hematology,* 7th ed. New York: McGraw-Hill; 2008. http://www.access medicine.com/resourceTOC.aspx?resourceID=69.

Linker CA. Blood. In: McPhee SJ, Papadakis MA, Tierney LM Jr. (Eds.), *Current Medical Diagnosis and Treatment,* 46th ed. New York: McGraw-Hill; 2007, pp. 493–547.

Medicinenet.com. Medical Dictionary. http://www.medterms.com/script/main/hp.asp.

Myeloid Leukemias, Myelodysplasia, and Myeloproliferative Syndromes. In: Kasper DL, Braunwald E, Fauci AS, Hauser SL, Longo DL, Jameson JL (Eds.), *Harrison's Manual of Medicine,* 16th ed. New York: McGraw-Hill; 2005, pp. 290–296.

National Cancer Institute. Chronic Myelogenous Leukemia Treatment (PDQ®). http://www.cancer.gov/cancertopics/pdq/treatment/CML.

*Stedman's Online Medical Dictionary.* http://www.stedmans.com/.

Wetzler M, Byrd JC, Bloomfield CD. Acute and Chronic Myeloid Leukemia. In: Fauci AS, Braunwald E, Kasper DL, Hauser SL, Longo DL, Jameson JL, Loscalzo J (Eds.), *Harrisons Online.* 2008. http://www.accessmedicine.com/content.aspx?aID =2891657.

# Chapter 8

# Hemophilia

## CHAPTER OBJECTIVES

✓ Describe the etiology and various forms of hemophilia.
✓ Detail phenotypic features, symptoms, and physical examination findings associated with hemophilia.
✓ Discuss variable expressivity of genes.
✓ Identify bleeding disorders associated with hemophilia.
✓ Review current diagnosis, treatment, and surveillance recommendations for hemophilia.

**Hemophilia** is a bleeding disorder caused by mutations in the F8 or F9 genes, which encode the coagulation proteins factor VIII and factor IX, respectively. Both of these factors play key roles in the blood clotting cascade (**Figure 8-1**). An F8 mutation resulting in a factor VIII deficiency manifests as **hemophilia A** or "classic hemophilia." An F9 mutation causes a factor IX deficiency and is designated as **hemophilia B** or "Christmas

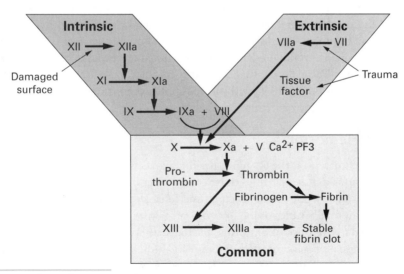

**Figure 8-1** Coagulation cascade.
*Source:* Reproduced with permission of Gordon M. Kirby, Ontario Veterinary College at the University of Guelph.

Table 8-1  **Classification of Hemophilia A and B by Normal Coagulation Factor Activity (Factor VIII and Factor IX) and Associated Clinical Findings**

| Classification | Percent Normal Factor Activity* | Associated Clinical Findings |
|---|---|---|
| Severe | < 1% | Spontaneous joint and muscle bleeding; post-trauma and postoperative bleeding |
| Moderate | 1% to 5% | Bleeding in joints and muscles due to minor trauma; postoperative bleeding |
| Mild | 5% to 40% | Postoperative and mild trauma bleeding |

*Reference range for normal clotting activity is 50% to 150%.
*Source:* Data from National Center for Biotechnology Information. U.S. National Library of Medicine. National Institute of Health. Available at http://eutils.wip.ncbi.nlm.nih.gov/bookshelf/br.fcgi?book=gene&part=hemo-a. Accessed January 19, 2010.

disease." Both F8 and F9 mutations are inherited in an **X-linked recessive** pattern, with mostly males being affected. Both types of hemophilia occur worldwide across all races. Approximately 1 in 4000 males is affected with hemophilia A, whereas hemophilia B is not as common and has an incidence of approximately 1 in 20,000 males.

Clinically, these two disorders are indistinguishable from each other. Both types of hemophilia present with spontaneous bleeding into the joints (**hemarthroses**), bleeding into muscles, and variable degrees of prolonged or abnormal bleeding in other soft tissues. Postoperative and traumatic bleeding may occur depending on the severity of the disease. Hemophilia is classified as mild, moderate, or severe based on the amount of normal coagulation factor activity (**Table 8-1**). Initial laboratory findings include a prolonged activated partial thromboplastin time (APTT) with normal prothrombin time (PT), normal bleeding time, and normal fibrinogen levels. The diagnosis is made by specific factor assays.

## Genetics of Hemophilia

Under normal circumstances, the F8 gene provides instructions for making factor VIII. In hemophilia A, various mutations in F8 cause the production of abnormal factor VIII proteins, which cannot carry out their expected functions. Depending on the specific mutation, the levels of normally functioning or active protein will vary; clinical manifestations are directly related to the amount of normal protein activity (Table 8-1). The F9 gene provides the instructions for making protein factor IX. In hemophilia B, various mutations in F9 cause production of abnormal factor IX proteins, which results in clinical manifestations similar to hemophilia A.

Both factor VIII and factor IX are integral components of the extrinsic coagulation pathway (Figure 8-1). These two proteins work in conjunction with other components of the blood to promote clotting and stop bleeding (**hemostasis**). Hemostasis also involves the action of platelets at the site of injury and the formation of a fibrin clot in a process known as **coagulation**. Coagulation is the chemical reaction that occurs among the various coagulation factors that results in a stable fibrin clot. When an injury occurs, blood clots form to seal off damaged blood vessels, thereby preventing further blood loss. In hemophilia, the coagulation factors are altered and are unable to mediate reactions in the coagulation cascade (Figure 8-1). As a result, clots do not form properly in response to an injury and abnormal bleeding occurs.

Because hemophilia A and hemophilia B are inherited in an X-linked recessive pattern, the mutated gene is located on the X chromosome. As we know, the sex chromosomes X and Y are distributed as XX in females and XY in males. Because males have only one X chromosome, only one mutated gene causes disease expression in them. In contrast, females have two X chromosomes, so the mutation must be present in both copies of the gene to cause the disorder in them. Therefore, males are affected by X-linked recessive disorders in greater frequency than females.

In X-linked recessive inheritance, females with one altered copy of the gene in each cell are considered to be **carriers**. A carrier female can pass the altered gene to her children, but generally does not express the disease herself. Some carrier females do manifest a mild disease expression. Because males pass only the Y chromosome on to their male offspring, hemophilia is not inherited from father to son.

## Diagnosis

Because hemophilia slows the blood clotting process, affected persons often present with prolonged bleeding after injury, surgery, or tooth extraction. Severity of symptoms is often variable (Table 8-1)—a phenomenon referred to as **variable expressivity**. In **severe hemophilia**, heavy bleeding can occur without any obvious trauma—a situation called **spontaneous bleeding**. Individuals with this type of hemophilia are usually diagnosed shortly after birth. Serious complications can result from bleeding into the weight-bearing joints and muscles as well as into the brain or internal organs. The joints most commonly affected are the knees, ankles, and elbows. Blood irritates the synovial lining of the affected joint and can lead to limited movement of the joint. Gastrointestinal bleeding is the most frequent cause of internal bleeding. Mild head trauma can also cause unusual bleeding and lead to a collection of blood under the skull, known as a **cephalohematoma**.

**Moderate hemophilia** may also present with hemarthoses or deep-tissue **hematomas** due to minor trauma or as postoperative bleeding. Persons with moderate hemophilia are typically diagnosed before 6 years of age. **Mild hemophilia** does not involve spontaneous bleeding and may become apparent only when abnormal bleeding occurs following surgery or a serious injury. Persons with mild hemophilia are frequently diagnosed later in life.

Other findings that vary with degree of severity of hemophilia include the propensity for excessive bleeding during menses (**menorrhagia**). Unexplained gastrointestinal or genitourinary bleeding may also occur. Prolonged nosebleeds that are recurrent over time, are bilateral, and are not elicited by trauma are often present. Prolonged oozing or bleeding after initial cessation of bleeding due to tooth extraction, buccal mucosa injury, or circumcision is common.

While a positive family history is helpful in making the diagnosis of hemophilia, it is important to note that approximately 25% of hemophiliacs do not present with a known family history. This may be attributed to very mild clinical manifestations or **de novo mutations** of the F8 or F9 gene. De novo mutations first occur in the affected person.

## Genetic Testing and Counseling

All individuals with a suspected bleeding disorder should undergo coagulation screening consisting of an APTT measurement, a PT measurement, a bleeding time measurement, and a platelet count.

The APTT measurement evaluates the intrinsic pathway of the coagulation cascade (Figure 8-1) and is the best individual screening test for coagulation disorders. It is most sensitive in patients with a clinical history of bleeding such as in moderate to severe hemophilia; it is less sensitive in those persons without clinical manifestations as in mild hemophilia. The APTT test is also clinically useful to monitor heparin therapy and to detect clotting inhibitors. The PT measurement evaluates the extrinsic pathway of the coagulation cascade and is clinically useful in monitoring long-term anticoagulant therapy with Coumadin (warfarin) as well as in evaluation of liver function and extrinsic factor disorders.

Neither PT nor APTT can differentiate between factor deficiencies or the presence of specific factor inhibitors such as anti-factor VIII. It is also important to note that low to normal clotting activity in these screening tests does not completely rule out the presence of hemophilia A. For these reasons, specific coagulation **factor assays** must be performed. Any person with a lifelong history of bleeding should have these coagulation factor assays performed, regardless of the results of the screening tests. Estrogens, oral contraceptives, epinephrine, **desmopressin acetate**, and vigorous exercise can all increase the levels of factors VIII and IX. Decreases in circulating factor VIII and IX may be due to in vivo consumption, such as occurs in **disseminated intravascular coagulation**.

The platelet count is most often a component of the complete blood count, but may also be ordered as a single test. It is useful to rule out bleeding disorders due to *quantitative* platelet disorders or **thrombocytopenia**. By comparison, the bleeding time is the best screening test for platelet function disorders. It is prolonged in **von Willebrand's disease** and in *qualitative* platelet disorders.

Once a specific **factor deficiency** is confirmed, attempts to identify specific mutations should be made. This effort begins with targeted mutation analysis for the two most common mutations (gene inversions) detected in the majority of severe hemophiliacs. Mutations in mild to moderate disease tend to be **missense mutations**, whereas **deletions** are associated with a poorer response to therapy. Specific mutations in each category correlate with severity of disease as well as response to **factor replacement therapy**.

Due to the X-linked inheritance pattern of hemophilia A and B, the carrier status of the mother determines the risk of transmitting the faulty genes to the siblings of the affected person. The identified affected person is known as the **proband**. Females who are carriers have a 50% chance per pregnancy of passing along the F8 mutation. As mentioned earlier, males who inherit the mutation will be affected, whereas females who inherit the mutation will be carriers. Affected males will transmit the mutation to all of their daughters but to none of their sons. When families in which some members have hemophilia are identified, it is important to construct an accurate pedigree, as this information will be helpful when counseling other family members.

## Management and Treatment

The recommended initial evaluation for patients newly diagnosed with hemophilia A or B should include identification of the specific mutation, a personal history of bleeding, family history of bleeding, a thorough musculoskeletal evaluation, associated disease screenings, and baseline laboratory tests. Identification of the specific mutations can aid in predicting the severity of disease, the development of factor inhibitors, and related immune tolerance. A history of personal and familial bleeding tendencies can also predict the severity of the disease. A complete examination of joints and muscles contributes to the estimation of disease severity given that hemarthroses and deep-tissue hematomas tend to occur more frequently with increasing disease severity. Screening for hepatitis A, hepatitis B, hepatitis C, and HIV is recommended for individuals who received blood or blood products such as **clotting factor** concentrates prior to 1985.

Referral to **hemophilia treatment centers** has been shown to be beneficial to patients with hemophilia, as evidenced by the lower mortality rates for those enrolled in such programs versus those who are not enrolled. These centers constitute a group of federally funded hospitals that specialize in coagulation disorders; care is delivered by teams that include a hematologist, nurse, social worker, and physical therapist, who work together to deliver comprehensive care by providing education, genetic counseling, and laboratory testing to patients and families. Centers may be located through the National Hemophilia Foundation (www.hemophilia.org).

Young children with hemophilia require assessment every 6 to 12 months. For persons receiving factor VIII concentrates, it is recommended that they initially be assessed at 3- to 6-month intervals and then annually once therapy is well established. Any individual with a milder form of hemophilia needs periodic assessment every 2 to 3 years. Screening is also recommended prior to any type of invasive surgery.

Treatment of bleeding manifestations for severe disease includes intravenous infusions of factor VIII concentrate within an hour of the onset of bleeding. Patients can be trained to administer these intravenous products at home. Nasal desmopressin or factor VIII concentrate may be used in mild to moderate disease. Prevention of bleeding episodes and complications should focus on reducing the risk of injury and precipitating events. For children, these guidelines include restrictions on specific physical activities such as contact sports. At the same time, it is important to recommend regular exercise to strengthen muscles and protect joints. Chronic joint disease may also be ameliorated by early recognition of hemarthroses. Other circumstances to be avoided prior to treatment include elective surgeries such as circumcision, intramuscular injections, dental procedures, and ingestion of aspirin or products containing aspirin.

Two major complications associated with factor replacement therapy are transfusion-transmitted infection and development of factor antibodies. Hemophiliacs treated prior to 1986 are at increased risk for the development of blood-borne infection. In particular, hepatitis A, hepatitis B, hepatitis C, and HIV infection have been associated with factor replacement therapy in patients who received human-derived blood products before viral testing and protein purification became a routine part of development of blood products. Fortunately, the incidence of transfusion-related infection has decreased with the development of recombinant factor concentrates and greater ability to eradicate viruses from the plasma-derived products. Recombinant factor concentrates do not contain any human-derived proteins.

Antibodies that develop in patients in response to factor replacement therapy are known as **factor inhibitors**. The risk of developing these antibodies is greatest during the initial treatment for hemophilia, when the body recognizes the factor infusion as "foreign" and mounts an immune response. Recently, gene therapy clinical trials for hemophilia A and B were discontinued. In these trials, patients were not able to achieve factor expression in quantities great enough to ameliorate disease symptoms. Complications also developed in several patients.

## Associated Syndromes

**Hemophilia B Leyden** is a rare variant of hemophilia B inherited in an X-linked pattern. This bleeding disorder is characterized by an altered developmental expression of blood coagulation factor IX and is associated with a variety of single-point mutations in the F9 gene. Affected individuals experience episodes of excessive bleeding in childhood, but have few bleeding problems after puberty.

Rarely, hemophilia may be acquired instead of inherited. **Acquired hemophilia** presents with the same clinical manifestations of inherited hemophilia, but usually first appears in adulthood. This condition is caused by the production of **autoantibody**, which inactivates coagulation factor VIII (acquired hemophilia A) or IX (acquired hemophilia B). The production of autoantibody has been associated with pregnancy, immune system disorders, cancer, and allergic reactions to certain drugs. In many cases, the etiology is not discovered.

Von Willebrand's disease is a bleeding disorder associated with low factor VIII activity in which von Willebrand factor (vWF), a blood protein, is either missing or does not function properly. This mutation is most frequently inherited in an autosomal dominant pattern with variable penetrance, although three rare subtypes show autosomal recessive inheritance patterns. Because it can be inherited by both men and women equally, von Willebrand's disease is the most common heritable bleeding disorder. **Acquired von Willebrand's disease** usually develops late in life and is caused by the development of antibodies that attack and destroy vWF. **Bleeding diatheses** that present with a prolonged APTT (with or without clinical manifestations) may be differentiated based on follow-up testing. Because of the complexity of these conditions and the increased risk of bleeding associated with them, referral to a hematologist is recommended whenever they are suspected.

Factor XI deficiency—also known as plasma thromboplastin antecedent (PTA) deficiency or **hemophilia C**—is second only to von Willebrand's disease among bleeding disorders affecting females. The incidence of factor XI deficiency is 1 in 100,000. This disease follows an autosomal recessive pattern of inheritance and occurs more frequently among members of some ethnic groups. For example, in Ashkenazi Jews, the incidence is approximately 1 in 10,000. Several genetic changes are known to be associated with factor XI deficiency, each of which induces a variable effect on bleeding. Factor XI deficiency is usually diagnosed after injury-related bleeding. Symptoms are typically mild, and almost half of all patients are completely asymptomatic. Affected individuals do not experience spontaneous bleeding or hemarthroses, but may have bruising, nosebleeds, blood in their urine, and prolonged bleeding after childbirth. Most affected persons do not require treatment.

## Chapter Summary

- Hemophilia A ("classic hemophilia") is a bleeding disorder caused by mutations in the F8 gene, which encodes for factor VIII.

- Hemophilia B ("Christmas disease") is a bleeding disorder caused by mutations in the F9 gene, which encodes for factor IX.

- F8 and F9 gene mutations are inherited in an X-linked recessive pattern, with only males affected by the resulting hemophilia; females are carriers of the mutations but rarely develop the disease itself.

- Hemophiliacs frequently present with spontaneous bleeding into joints (hemarthroses) and muscles (hematomas), and experience variable degrees of prolonged or abnormal bleeding.

- Screening tests for hemophilia include prolonged activated partial thromboplastin time with normal prothrombin time, normal bleeding time, and normal fibrinogen levels.

- Diagnosis of hemophilia is made by specific factor assays.

- Evaluation of a person with newly diagnosed hemophilia A or B should include identification of the specific mutation, a personal history of bleeding, family history of bleeding, a thorough musculoskeletal evaluation, associated disease screenings, and baseline laboratory tests.

- Factor VIII concentrate and nasal desmopressin are used to treat bleeding episodes and for maintenance therapy.

## Key Terms

**Acquired hemophilia:** production of autoantibody that inactivates coagulation factors (VIII or IX) and results in the same clinical bleeding diathesis as occurs in inherited hemophilias.

**Acquired von Willebrand's disease:** a form of von Willebrand's disease that is not inherited but rather develops late in life. It is caused by the development of antibodies that attack and destroy a person's von Willebrand factor. This disease is commonly "acquired" in conjunction with another serious disease.

**Autoantibody:** a protein that attacks the body's own tissues.

**Bleeding diathesis:** a group of distinct conditions in which a person's body cannot properly develop a clot, resulting in an increased tendency for bleeding.

**Carrier:** a person (usually female) who can pass an altered gene to her children, but generally does not express the disease herself.

**Cephalohematoma:** a collection of blood under the skull due to an effusion of blood, usually as a result of trauma.

**Clotting factor:** any of several proteins that are involved in the blood coagulation process.

**Coagulation:** the chemical reaction mediated by coagulation factor proteins that results in a stable fibrin clot.

**De novo mutations:** mutations that are not inherited, but rather appear first in the affected individual.

**Deletion:** any spontaneous elimination of part of the normal genetic complement, whether cytogenetically visible (chromosomal deletion) or found by molecular techniques.

**Desmopressin acetate:** a synthetic hormone that increases factor VIII levels.

**Disseminated intravascular coagulation:** a condition of altered coagulation that results in consumption of clotting factors and platelets and yields a clinical presentation characterized by both excessive clotting and excessive bleeding.

**Factor assay:** a specialized lab test used to determine the level of circulating factor VIII or IX.

**Factor deficiency:** any of several rare disorders characterized by the complete absence or an abnormally low level of clotting factor in the blood.

**Factor inhibitors:** antibodies that develop in patients in response to factor replacement therapy.

**Factor replacement therapy:** replacement of a deficient clotting factor from another source (either human derived or recombinant) in an effort to stop or prevent abnormal bleeding.

**Hemarthroses:** bleeding into joints.

**Hematoma:** bleeding into soft tissue, such as muscle or visceral organs.

**Hemophilia:** a bleeding disorder in which a specific clotting factor protein—namely, factor VIII or IX—is missing or does not function normally.

**Hemophilia A:** a deficiency or absence of factor VIII; also been called "classic" hemophilia. It is the most common severe bleeding disorder.

**Hemophilia B:** a deficiency or absence of factor IX; also called "Christmas disease" after the first family that was identified with the condition.

**Hemophilia B Leyden:** a rare variant of hemophilia B inherited in an X-linked pattern.

**Hemophilia C:** a deficiency or absence of factor XI; more commonly known as plasma thromboplastin antecedent deficiency.

**Hemophilia treatment centers:** a group of federally funded hospitals that specialize in treating patients with coagulation disorders.

**Hemostasis:** the process by which the body stops bleeding.

**Menorrhagia:** excessive bleeding during the time of menses, in terms of either duration or volume, or both.

**Mild hemophilia:** a categorical term used to describe someone with a factor VIII or IX level ranging between 5% and 25% of normal blood levels.

**Missense mutation:** a mutation in which a base change or substitution results in a codon that causes insertion of a different amino acid into the growing polypeptide chain, giving rise to an altered protein.

**Moderate hemophilia:** a categorical term used to describe someone with a factor VIII or IX level ranging between 1% and 5% of normal blood levels.

**Proband:** an affected person as identified in a family pedigree.

**Severe hemophilia:** a categorical term used to describe someone with a factor VIII or IX level that is less than 1% of normal blood levels.

**Spontaneous bleeding:** heavy bleeding without history of trauma.

**Thrombocytopenia:** a condition in which an abnormally small number of platelets appear in the circulating blood.

**Variable expressivity:** variation in which the disease symptoms are present.

**Von Willebrand's disease:** a bleeding disorder in which von Willebrand factor, a blood protein, is either missing or does not function properly. It is the most common congenital bleeding disorder in the United States.

**X-linked recessive:** recessive inheritance pattern of alleles at loci on the X chromosome that do not undergo crossing over during male meiosis.

## Chapter Review Questions

1. Hemophilia is a bleeding disorder caused by mutations in the _____ or _____ genes.

2. Generally, in an X-linked recessive pattern of inheritance, only _____ are affected.

3. A person with severe hemophilia often presents with _____, _____, and _____.

4. Screening test results consistent with hemophilia that warrant further evaluation include _____, _____, _____, _____, and _____.

5. Treatment for severe and moderate hemophilia includes _____.

## Resources

Bolton-Maggs PH, Pasi KJ. Haemophilias A and B. *Lancet.* 361:1801–1809; 2003.

Gene Reviews. www.genetests.org.

Genetics Home Reference. ghr.nlm.nih.gov.

National Heart, Lung and Blood Institute. www.nlm.nih.gov.

National Hemophilia Foundation. www.hemophilia.org.

Pierce GF, Lillicrap D, Pipe SW, Vandendriessche T. Gene therapy, Bioengineered Clotting Factors and Novel Technologies for Hemophilia Treatment. *Journal of Thrombosis and Haemostasis.* 5:901–906; 2007.

*Stedman's Online Medical Dictionary.* www.stedmans.com.

# Chapter 9

# Sickle Cell Disease

## CHAPTER OBJECTIVES

✓ Describe the etiology and various forms of sickle cell disease.
✓ Detail the symptoms associated with sickle cell disease.
✓ Discuss novel property mutations, heterozygote advantage, and ethnic variation of allelic frequency.
✓ Review the current treatment recommendations for sickle cell disease.

Sickle cell disease results from a **point mutation** in the hemoglobin beta (HBB) gene that causes a single change in the amino acid sequence and results in substitution of valine for glutamine in the β subunit of hemoglobin. This change confers a new property on hemoglobin, but does not alter how this protein transports oxygen in the blood. Such a change in a gene is known as a **novel property mutation**.

Normal adult hemoglobin is designated hemoglobin A (HbA), whereas adult sickle hemoglobin is designated as hemoglobin S (HbS). Hemoglobin S is correlated with lower rates of mortality among carriers who are of African and Mediterranean descent, because the HbS allele decreases the risk of infection by malarial parasites endemic in those areas. This property is referred to as **heterozygote advantage**.

When red cells deoxygenate, the HbS chains are transformed into rigid polymers, which results in rigid, crescent-shaped red blood cells. These "sickled" cells are unable to flow freely through small vessels, which results in pain and ultimately vaso-occlusive infarctions in multiple organ systems. Pain, infections, and bone infarctions are hallmark clinical presentations of sickle cell disease, along with varying degrees of **anemia**. The vascular endothelium, white blood cells, inflammatory process, and coagulation cascade are also adversely affected.

## Genetics of Sickle Cell Disease

Sickle cell disease is inherited in an autosomal recessive pattern. Because recessive inheritance requires that both alleles be present for disease expression, both defective genes (SS) are needed for sickle cell disease to occur. When offspring inherit one recessive allele (S) and one normal allele (A), they become unaffected carriers (AS) (**Figure 9-1**). This heterozygous expression of HbS is known as **sickle cell trait**.

The overall prevalence of sickle cell disease in the United States is approximately 1 in 72,000 and varies by ethnic origin. Among African Americans, the incidence is about 1 in 500, whereas in Hispanic Americans the incidence is 1 in 1400. The sickle cell mutation

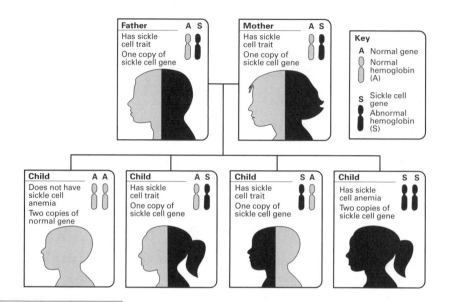

**Figure 9-1** Inheritance pattern of hemoglobin S.
*Source:* From National Heart, Lung, and Blood Institute, Disease and Conditions Index. Available at http://www.nhlbi.nih.gov/health/dci/Diseases/Sca/SCA_Causes.html. Accessed January 20, 2010.

is also more common among persons whose ancestry is geographically connected to sub-Saharan Africa, Cuba, South America, Central America, Saudi Arabia, India. and the Mediterranean regions—a phenomenon known as **ethnic variation of allelic frequency**. An estimated 2 million Americans carry the sickle cell trait.

## Phenotypic Features

The abnormal hemoglobin of sickle cell disease (SS) is detectable at birth. Consequently, all states in the United States now require newborn screening for HbS. Affected individuals who test negative on newborn screening or who bypass screening usually present with the disease within the first two years of life. Common presenting symptoms include failure to thrive, anemia, splenomegaly, multiple chronic infections, and swelling of the extremities resulting from vaso-occlusion. Patients who present much more acutely—that is, "in crisis"—may have severe abdominal pain, stroke, acute chest syndrome, renal necrosis, leg ulcers, priapism (a painful persistent erection), or loss of vision due to a massive vaso-occlusive infarction.

The clinical manifestations of sickle cell disease are related directly or indirectly to hemolysis and vaso-occlusion. Hemolysis contributes to chronic anemia and subsequent jaundice. Rapid red blood cell destruction increases bilirubin and can lead to cholelithiasis; it also predisposes affected patients to aplastic crisis. Vaso-occlusion can cause tissue ischemia distal to the obstruction and result in tissue death. The brain, lungs, kidneys, and glans penis are frequently affected by this kind of vaso-occlusive disease.

The spleen is particularly susceptible to ischemia, with frequent episodes of spleno-megaly being noted in patients with **hemoglobin SC disease**, whereas HbSS patients will undergo splenic auto-infarction during childhood. Hemoglobin SC disease occurs in people who have one copy of the gene for sickle cell disease and one copy of the gene for **hemoglobin C disease**. Symptoms associated with HbSC disease are similar to sickle cell disease, but tend to be milder in some patients.

Painful swelling of the hands and feet may be the earliest manifestation of sickle cell disease in infants and young children. Acute chest syndrome occurs when vascular occlusion and inflammation affect the small vessels of the bronchial tree. While the signs and symptoms of acute chest syndrome vary among patients, infiltrates may or may not be identified on chest x-ray, and patients may present with pain, respiratory illness, fever, and shortness of breath. Treatment of acute chest syndrome should be based on presenting clinical symptoms, given that accurate chest x-ray diagnosis will lag behind the clinical picture in many cases. The leading cause of death among adult patients with sickle cell disease is acute chest syndrome, although infection and fat emboli are also thought to play a role in bringing about this syndrome.

An acutely enlarged spleen with a hemoglobin level at least 2 g/dL below baseline are indicative of splenic sequestration of red blood cells. Low platelet count, abdominal pain, nausea, and vomiting may also be present. This presentation occurs most frequently in young children with sickle cell disease and may include a febrile illness.

When vessels in the brain become occluded, patients with sickle cell disease may present with acute stroke-like symptoms such as headache, hemiparesis, seizures, impaired speech, palsies involving cranial nerves, or mental status changes. The age range associated with stroke risk is bimodal—namely, children between the ages of 2 and 9 years and older adults are at greatest risk. In the absence of a stroke, smaller infarctions may lead to gradual cognitive changes in persons with sickle cell disease.

Priapism is a frequent occurrence in males with sickle cell disease and may cause permanent tissue damage and impotence if not treated. Other problems associated with reduced blood supply include avascular necrosis of the femoral and/or humeral head, renal failure, cardiomyopathies, delayed growth, and superficial ulcers of the lower extremities. Even though patients with sickle cell trait do not usually have clinical symptoms, under some circumstances a change in environmental conditions may lead to episodes of ischemia in these individuals. For example, exposures to high altitudes (such as in mountain hiking or flying in an unpressurized aircraft) and prolonged severe physical exertion can result in symptoms similar to those of sickle cell disease due to severe anoxia.

## Clinical Diagnosis and Testing

Sickle cell disease is suspected when a young child presents with painful swelling of the hands and feet, a condition that is also known as "hand–foot syndrome." Patients may also present with symptoms of anemia, infection, splenomegaly, or acute chest syndrome. Family history is helpful in establishing a working diagnosis.

The complete blood count (CBC) typically demonstrates a normocytic anemia with **target cells**. When hypoxemia is present, sickled cells are also reported. This finding should prompt the clinician to screen for HbS by using a solubility test. This test causes any HbS that is present to precipitate, but it does not differentiate between sickle cell disease and sickle cell trait because HbS is present in both states. Any screening test that is positive for HbS or other significant hemoglobinopathies in a newborn must be confirmed by 6 weeks of age. The presence of large quantities of HbS using hemoglobin electrophoresis is considered diagnostic for sickle cell disease. Similarly, electrophoresis is used to confirm sickle cell trait by identifying the presence of HbS, albeit in lower quantities than are present in sickle cell disease. Because of the high mortality rate associated with undiagnosed sickle cell disease in infants and young children, newborn screenings are now required for all infants born in a U.S. state or territory.

## Other Sickle Cell Disorders

Sickle cell disease exists in many forms, but HbSS is the most common type, followed by HbSC. Non-sickling beta hemoglobin disorders such as thalassemia can interact with a sickle cell disease mutation to cause clinically significant disease; these variants of sickle cell disease expression are known as sickle beta-plus thalassemia (HbSβ$^{+ \text{THAL}}$) and sickle beta-zero thalassemia (HbSβ$^{0 \text{THAL}}$) (**Table 9-1**).

## Management and Treatment

Management of sickle cell disease primarily focuses on prevention of crises and management of symptoms. Patients should be counseled to avoid precipitating activities that

**Table 9-1  Hemoglobin Distribution in Sickle Cell Syndromes**

| Genotype | Clinical Diagnosis (Phenotype) | Hb A[1] | Hb S[2] | Hb A2[3] | Hb F[4] |
|---|---|---|---|---|---|
| AA | Normal | 97–99% | 0 | 1–2% | < 1% |
| AS | Sickle trait | 60% | 40% | 1–2% | < 1% |
| SS | Sickle cell anemia | 0 | 86–98% | 1–3% | 5–15% |
| Sβ$^0$-thalassemia* | Sickle β-thalassemia | 0 | 70–80% | 3–5% | 10–20% |
| Sβ$^+$-thalassemia† | Sickle β-thalassemia | 10–20% | 60–75% | 3–5% | 10–20% |
| AS, α-thalassemia‡ | Sickle trait | 70–75% | 25–30% | 1–2% | < 1% |

1. Hb A = hemoglobin A (adult).
2. Hb S = hemoglobin S (sickle).
3. Hb A2 = hemoglobin A$^2$ (adult 2).
4. Hb F = hemoglobin F (fetal).
*Sβ$^{0 \text{THAL}}$ = sickle beta-zero thalassemia.
†Sβ$^{+ \text{THAL}}$ = sickle beta-plus thalassemia.
‡α-thalassemia = alpha thalassemia.

*Source:* Tierney LM, et al. *Current Medical Diagnosis & Treatment*, 45th ed; 2006, p. 1251. Copyright © The McGraw-Hill Companies, Inc. All rights reserved.

might lead to sickle cell crisis, such as dehydration, physical stress, infection, change in altitude, and prolonged exposure to extreme temperatures. Symptoms associated with crises are addressed specifically, and a pain management plan should be developed for this possibility, which may involve the use of opiates and other analgesics. Broad-spectrum antibiotics are indicated when the patient presents with fever. It is important that affected individuals stay current on immunizations (i.e., influenza, pneumonia). Furthermore, patients should be counseled to seek immediate medical attention for signs and symptoms of crises so as to prevent complications.

Surveillance is individualized, but laboratory tests routinely include annual CBC, reticulocyte count, iron status, liver enzymes, bilirubin, blood urea nitrogen, creatinine, and urinalysis. Doppler studies of the brain to detect areas of decreased or increased flow, chest x-rays, pulmonary function testing, gallbladder ultrasound, and echocardiogram may be indicated depending on the patient's status and age. Red blood cell transfusions can benefit patients with sickle cell disease by decreasing their risk of stroke, pulmonary hypertension, and painful crises. Conversely, repeated transfusions will result in iron overload, so iron and ferritin levels must be monitored closely and reduced before iron accumulates and causes permanent organ damage. Liver biopsy with iron dry-weight quantitation will provide the most accurate picture of the total body iron burden. Repeated or prolonged transfusion regimens can also result in alloimmunization, or the exposure to foreign antigens in the red blood cell unit. This condition results in circulating antibodies in the patient, making it more difficult to ensure future compatibility with donor red blood cell units.

Hydroxyurea is the most commonly prescribed therapy for sickle cell disease. It works by multiple mechanisms. First, it improves red blood cell survival by inducing production of fetal hemoglobin (HgF) that is resistant to sickling. Second, it lowers the white blood cell count and arrests inflammatory processes. Third, it metabolizes into nitric oxide, which acts as a vasodilator to help improve blood flow and reduce the risk of stroke. The use of hydroxyurea has been shown to reduce the number of painful episodes, acute chest syndrome, and transfusions as well as to improve overall survival among persons with sickle cell disease. Allogeneic transplant is the only available curative treatment for sickle cell disease, but few patients have a suitable donor available. When a suitable donor is available, stem cell transplant has been reported to produce a disease-free survival rate as high as 85%, with the best outcomes reported in pediatric patients.

## Genetic Counseling

When counseling high-risk individuals, it is important to consider other beta-chain disorders that may contribute to sickle cell disease. The carrier states for hemoglobinopathies other than HbS may be unknown in those persons who have never been screened for these abnormalities. The optimal time for counseling is during preconception family planning. When patients present after conception, early testing is important. Prenatal diagnosis for those at increased risk is possible through amniocentesis. However, because there is wide variation in clinical presentations among affected individuals, it is impossible to predict the extent or outcome of sickle cell disease.

## Chapter Summary

- Sickle cell disease is caused by a mutation in the hemoglobin beta (HBB) gene, leading to a single change in amino acid sequence.
- Sickle cell disease typically presents in early childhood in the United States, identified through required newborn screening.
- The diagnosis of sickle cell disease is made from hemoglobin electrophoresis and other confirmatory testing after a positive screening test.
- Sickle cell trait is usually clinically silent but it may produce symptoms when exacerbated by hypoxia.
- Mortality in sickle cell disease is related to the number and severity of crises; crises may lead to stroke, acute chest syndrome, complications of anemia, and infections.
- Surveillance guidelines are individualized depending on the patient's age and disease status.
- Hydroxyurea improves overall survival and reduces symptoms.

## Key Terms

**Anemia:** any condition in which the number of red blood cells per cubic millimeter (mm³), the amount of hemoglobin in 100 mL of blood, and/or the volume of packed red blood cells per 100 mL of blood are less than normal.

**Ethnic variation of allelic frequency:** a situation which frequency of mutated alleles is higher among certain ethnic groups than in others.

**Hemoglobin C disease:** a type of hemoglobin-related disease characterized by episodes of abdominal and joint pain, an enlarged spleen, and mild jaundice, but no severe crises. This disease occurs mostly in African Americans, who may show few symptoms of its presence.

**Hemoglobin SC disease:** a type of hemoglobin-related disease that occurs in people who have one copy of the gene for sickle cell disease and one copy of the gene for hemoglobin C disease.

**Heterozygote advantage:** a mutated allele at the same locus as a normal allele that confers the advantage of protection against a disease and increases survival.

**Novel property mutation:** a mutation that confers a new property on the protein product.

**Point mutation:** the alteration of a single nucleotide to a different nucleotide.

**Sickle cell trait:** the heterozygous state of the gene for hemoglobin S in sickle cell anemia.

**Target cell:** an erythrocyte with a dark center surrounded by a light band that is encircled by a darker ring; thus it resembles a shooting target.

## Chapter Review Questions

1. When the offspring inherit one affected recessive allele (S) and one normal allele (A), they become unaffected carriers (AS) and are said to have _____.

2. The mutation that causes sickle cell disease is more common among persons whose ancestry is geographically connected to the following geographic regions: _____, _____, _____, _____, _____, _____, and _____.

3. The chance of two parents with sickle cell trait (HbAS) have a child with sickle cell disease (HbSS) is _____; this is described as an _____ pattern of inheritance.

4. Clinical findings that raise suspicion for sickle cell disease in a young child include _____, _____, _____, and _____.

5. A mutation that confers a new property on the protein is called a _____ mutation.

## Resources

American College of Medical Genetics. www.acmg.net.

American Society of Hematology. http://www.hematology.org/.

Ashley-Koch A, Yang Q, Olney RS. Sickle Hemoglobin (*Hb S*) Allele and Sickle Cell Disease: A HuGE Review. *American Journal of Epidemiology.* 151(9):839–845; 2000.

Gene Reviews. www.genetests.org.

Genetics Home Reference. http://ghr.nlm.nih.gov/.

Jorde LB, Carey JC, Bamshad MJ, White RL. *Medical Genetics,* 3rd ed. Philadelphia: Mosby; 2006.

Linker CA. Blood. In: Tierney LM Jr., McPhee SJ, Papadakis MA (Eds.), *Current Medical Diagnosis and Treatment,* 45th ed. New York: McGraw-Hill; 2006, pp. 481–535.

*The Merck Manual* Online Medical Library. http://www.merck.com/mmhe/sec14/ch172/ch172h.html.

National Heart, Lung and Blood Institute. http://www.nhlbi.nih.gov/.

Sickle Cell Information Center. http://www.scinfo.org/.

*Stedman's Online Medical Dictionary.* http://www.stedmans.com/.

Tietz NW. *Clinical Guide to Laboratory Tests,* 3rd ed. Philadelphia: W. B. Saunders; 1995.

# Chapter 10

# Hemochromatosis

## CHAPTER OBJECTIVES

✓ Describe etiology and forms of hemochromatosis.
✓ Detail phenotypic features, symptoms, and physical examination findings associated with hemochromatosis.
✓ Discuss sex-influenced phenotype, variable expressivity, and penetrance.
✓ Review current treatment and surveillance recommendations for hemochromatosis.

**Hereditary hemochromatosis** (type 1 HHC) is an autosomal recessive disorder that is caused by a single mutation in the HFE gene. This mutation causes increased intestinal absorption of iron and results in increased iron storage in body tissues such as those found in the liver, pancreas, skin, heart, and other organs—a phenomenon referred to as HFE-associated hereditary hemochromatosis (HFE-HHC). In the United States, approximately 1 in 250 Caucasian persons are homozygous for the HFE mutation, while another 1 in 10 are heterozygous. Thus HFE-HHC is the most common single-gene disorder among Caucasians in the United States. This disorder is approximately 10 times more common in males than in females. As mentioned in Chapter 1, heterozygotes for recessive disorders are known as **carriers**.

## Phenotypic Features

Because persons with HHC absorb excess iron over a period of years, clinical evidence of disease does not typically present until the affected individual is 40 years of age or older. The average body stores approximately 4 grams of total iron in various forms. In symptomatic individuals, total body iron ranges between 15 and 40 grams—that is, 4 to 10 times more iron than is required for proper body functioning. Clinical manifestations of HHC are related to total body iron levels, but begin with increased serum iron concentration and then lead to increased liver iron stores.

Accumulation of iron over time results in tissue injury and ultimately progression to **cirrhosis** of the liver and other organ failure. Cirrhosis is a degenerative liver disease characterized by formation of fibrous tissue and scarring along with inhibition of normal cellular function. The most common presenting symptoms in early stages of this disease are fatigue, joint aches, and male sexual dysfunction (impotence). Many patients will have abnormal liver function tests at this stage in the disease's course. Less common findings include an enlarged liver (**hepatomegaly**), abdominal pain, diabetes mellitus, heart murmurs, conduction disturbances noted on electrocardiogram, hypothyroidism, arthritis,

Table 10-1 **Clinical Presentation of Hereditary Hemochromatosis**

| Reversible Manifestations | Permanent Manifestations |
| --- | --- |
| Cardiomyopathy | Cirrhosis |
| Arrhythmia | Hepatocellular carcinoma |
| Abdominal pain, hepatomegaly, abnormal liver function tests | Hypogonadism |
| | Diabetes mellitus |
| Skin hyperpigmentation | Hypothyroidism |
| Infection | Arthritis/pseudogout |

and hyperpigmented skin. In the past, hemochromatosis was referred to as "bronze diabetes" due to the common occurrence of insulin resistance and bronze skin coloration. In recent decades, this presentation has become increasingly rare.

Expression of disease symptoms varies among individuals with the same genetic mutation, with these variations reflecting differences in **penetrance** and **variable expressivity**. Penetrance describes the proportion of individuals carrying a particular mutation who express an associated, observable trait. It indicates the likelihood that symptoms will develop in the presence of a mutation. Variable expressivity describes the wide variation in types of symptoms and severity of symptoms observed when disease expression is present. However, disease expression can be accelerated by conditions causing decreased liver function, such as alcohol abuse and hepatitis. Many manifestations of HHC resolve after treatment; others are not reversible (**Table 10-1**).

Phenotypic expression of HHC is found in both men and women, but is clinically expressed at 10 times greater frequency in men. The lower incidence of clinical expression in women is attributed to a lower dietary iron intake as well as iron loss associated with menstruation. This difference in disease expression by gender is an example of a **sex-influenced phenotype**.

## Genetics of HFE-Associated Hemochromatosis

The HFE gene associated with type 1 HHC is located on the short arm of chromosome 6. Mutations caused by a single amino acid substitution are known as **point mutations**; the two most common point mutations in the HFE gene are designated as C282Y and H63D. Although iron overload may occur with any HFE mutation, the greatest risk is conferred with being homozygous for the C282Y mutation.

## Diagnosis

The diagnosis of HHC requires clinical findings as well as laboratory studies. Because iron absorption occurs along a continuum, clinical manifestations vary by stage and degree of iron overload. Patients rarely initially present with advanced end-organ damage secondary to iron overload. Instead, affected individuals are more frequently diagnosed based on serological evidence of HFE-HHC, which includes elevated **transferrin** saturation and serum ferritin concentrations. Elevated serum liver enzymes, abdominal pain in the right upper quadrant, fatigue, and arthralgias are frequent complaints at this stage of the disease course. Factors that raise clinical suspicion of advanced iron overload include hepatomegaly, hepatic cirrhosis, hepatocellular carcinoma, diabetes mellitus, cardiomyopathy, hypogonadism, arthritis, and hyperpigmented skin. These issues may be discovered through physical examination findings, a positive personal history, or a positive family history.

Under usual circumstances, 70% of iron is distributed in the body as hemoglobin in red blood cells. The remaining 30% is present as free serum iron, ferritin, and hemosiderin. While most iron is obtained from the diet (i.e., through consumption of red meat), only 10% of all ingested iron is absorbed in the small intestine and transported to the blood. In the blood, iron is bound to the protein transferrin and then transported to the bone marrow, where it can be incorporated into hemoglobin molecules.

Laboratory studies for HHC typically include **serum iron levels**, **serum ferritin levels**, **total iron binding capacity (TIBC)**, and **transferrin saturation levels (Table 10-2)**. Serum iron identifies the amount of free iron that was recently absorbed from the diet, but before it has become bound to transferrin. Normal serum iron levels are often detected in HHC due to storage of the majority of iron in other forms. The serum ferritin level is a measurement of the amount of circulating iron bound to transferrin. The TIBC is a measure of all proteins that are available to bind iron. It indirectly measures the amount of transferrin present, whereas transferrin saturation represents the portion of transferrin bound to iron. This value is determined by dividing serum iron by the TIBC:

$$\text{Transferrin saturation (\%)} = \frac{\text{Serum iron level} \times 100\%}{\text{TIBC}}$$

Approximately 80% of all persons with an HFE mutation will have a fasting transferrin saturation of 50% to 60%, with higher values often observed in males. Transferrin saturation

Table 10-2 **Summary of Expected Serum Iron Values in HFE-Hereditary Hemochromatosis Patients**

| Assay | Assay Explanation | Result |
|---|---|---|
| Serum iron | Free iron in serum | Normal to increased |
| Serum ferritin | Iron bound to transferrin in serum | Increased |
| Serum transferrin saturation | Transferrin bound to iron in serum | Increased |
| Total iron binding capacity | Transferrin available to bind iron | Normal to decreased |

*Source:* Tietz NW. *Clinical Guide to Laboratory Tests*, 3rd ed. 1995.

rates are not related to age, however, and they do not correlate with disease symptomology or severity. Because this value is directly correlated with the iron burden, serum transferrin has a high sensitivity and specificity for HHC: A threshold transferrin saturation of 45% is sensitive for detecting HFE-HHC. Elevated transferrin saturation levels are typically the earliest phenotypic manifestation of HHC, preceding clinical manifestations of the disease.

Serum ferritin levels increase progressively over time in individuals with HFE-HHC. Elevated serum ferritin levels are sensitive predictors of disease, but are not specific because serum ferritin may be elevated by any inflammatory process. Thus this biomarker is referred to as an **acute-phase reactant**. Serum ferritin tends to increase or decrease in the same direction as iron stores and provides a rough estimate of total body iron. In persons with HHC, a serum ferritin threshold of greater than 1000 μg/L is predictive of cirrhosis, **myelodysplastic syndromes**, and **aplastic anemia**. Underproduction of a single type of blood cell produced in the bone marrow is categorized as a myelodysplastic syndrome, in contrast to aplastic anemia, which involves total bone marrow failure and is characterized by a decrease in all blood cells. When serum ferritin is elevated above 2500 μg/L for a prolonged period, it is associated with an increased incidence of **cardiomyopathy**.

It should be noted that if both transferrin saturation and serum ferritin are elevated, these findings have a higher combined sensitivity and specificity in supporting the diagnosis of HHC than using either value alone. If only one of these values is elevated, liver biopsy is considered to be the "gold standard" for diagnosis and assessing the amount of fibrosis. Similar to HHC, cirrhosis is an independent risk factor for the development of hepatocellular carcinoma. The risk of developing hepatocellular carcinoma is approximately 200 times greater in patients with *both* HHC and cirrhosis. A serum ferritin level greater than 1000 μg/L is the recommended threshold for performing a liver biopsy due to its significant association with advanced fibrosis.

When serum iron studies are inconclusive, a liver biopsy can establish a definitive diagnosis by quantifying liver iron levels. Patients with HHC typically have a hepatic iron concentration exceeding 10,000 μg/g of liver tissue. The hepatic iron index takes into account the age of the patient because iron stores tend to diminish with increasing age:

$$\text{Hepatic iron index} = \text{Liver iron (μmol)} \div \text{Patient age (years)}$$

A hepatic iron index greater than 2 is diagnostic of HHC, whereas a hepatic iron index less than 2 is consistent with causes other than HHC—for example, alcoholic liver disease.

## Genetic Testing and Counseling

The wide availability of HFE gene testing may eventually eliminate the need for liver biopsy. This testing is performed by **polymerase chain reaction (PCR)** using a whole blood sample, which makes it relatively affordable compared to other genetic tests. This technique is very useful for screening family members of an affected person.

Although most parents of HHC-affected individuals are heterozygous for the HFE mutation and do not develop the disease themselves, the iron studies detailed previously may also be used to screen for disease expression. However, it is important to note that carriers may have abnormal test results. Each sibling of an affected person has a 25% chance of being affected and a 50% risk of being a carrier. Because the disease does not become manifest until later in adult life, identifying those persons at risk for iron over-load may help to ameliorate complications and improve overall survival. These factors make it reasonable to screen all adult patients with any family history of iron overload, personal history of chronic liver disease, or signs and symptoms of HHC. Once a diagnosis of HHC is established in an individual, all adult family members should be assessed for evidence of iron overload. Pediatric screening is not recommended, however.

## Management and Treatment

Treatment is generally initiated based on the presence of clinical symptoms. **Therapeutic phlebotomy**, which involves the removal of a portion of the affected individual's blood volume, is the treatment of choice for iron overload in patients with a serum ferritin greater than 1000 µg/L. This recommendation reflects the ease of undertaking this therapy as well as its low cost and effectiveness in decreasing the iron burden. Therapeutic phlebotomy is routinely initiated when clinical symptoms of HHC are present, with 400 to 500 mL of blood being removed on each occasion. This volume of whole blood with a normal hematocrit of about 40% effectively removes 160 to 200 mg of iron. Weekly phlebotomy is performed until the serum ferritin level reaches approximately 50 µg/L and the TIBC is less than 50% or until the individual's hematocrit is 75% of baseline hematocrit. Continued measurement of serum ferritin levels should be performed to monitor the therapeutic effects of phlebotomy. Men typically require the removal of twice the volume of blood as women need. Once these target levels are achieved, maintenance phlebotomy may be performed four times annually in men and twice annually in women to prevent the re-accumulation of iron. Serum ferritin levels should be reassessed at these same follow-up intervals.

Liver transplant is the only treatment for HFE-HHC patients with end-stage liver disease. Unfortunately, post-transplant survival in this patient population is generally poor.

Dietary management should involve avoidance of iron-containing supplements and limited intake of foods that are high in iron. Consumption of excessive amounts of vitamin C should also be avoided—this water-soluble vitamin increases absorption of dietary iron. Patients with impaired hepatic function should avoid drinking alcohol because iron and alcohol have **synergistic hepatotoxic effects**.

Screening guidelines for HHC patients with confirmed cirrhosis include **hepatic ultrasound** and serum **alpha-fetoprotein (AFP)** testing. Hepatic ultrasound can detect solid tumors or cystic changes in the liver and is recommended due to the increased risk of hepatic cancers such as primary hepatocellular carcinoma (also known as **hepatoma**). Although they are a nonspecific marker, serum AFP levels are increased in approximately

90% of all patients with hepatomas. Generally, the level of AFP is directly proportional to tumor burden. Other common causes of elevated serum AFP in HHC patients include cirrhosis and chronic active **hepatitis**.

## Associated Syndromes

Primary iron overload syndromes are defined by an increased absorption of iron from a normal diet. Most are types of HHC that are unrelated to mutations in the HFE gene. For example, juvenile HHC (type 2 HHC) results from mutations in the HJV or HAMP gene. Although this disease has characteristics that are similar to those of HFE-HHC, its clinical manifestations are more severe and appear at an earlier age. TFR2-related HHC (type 3 HHC) is caused by mutations in the TFR-2 gene; incidence of this disease is higher in certain Italian populations. Like type 2 HHC, type 3 HHC presents at an earlier age but is not as severe as type 2. Both types 1 and 2 HHC are inherited in an autosomal recessive pattern. Ferroportin-related iron overload (type 4 HHC) is caused by mutations in the *SLC40A1* gene and is inherited in an autosomal dominant pattern. African (Bantu) iron overload is a predisposition to iron overload that is exacerbated by excessive intake of iron. Neonatal hemochromatosis is a severe iron overload syndrome that begins in utero and is often fatal. To date, no specific mutations or inheritance patterns have been identified for neonatal hemochromatosis.

Secondary iron overload syndromes include conditions or diseases that result in specific tissue damage and iron overload from increased iron intake. Culprits include iron that is either ingested in dietary forms or absorbed from iron cookware as well as other sources of iron such as intramuscular supplements or blood transfusions. Persons at risk for secondary iron overload syndromes include individuals with alcoholic liver disease, viral hepatitis, porphyria cutanea tarda, rheumatoid arthritis, sickle cell disease, thalassemia, and other chronic anemias that require transfusion therapy.

## Chapter Summary

- Hereditary hemochromatosis is caused by mutations in the HFE gene and is inherited in an autosomal recessive pattern.
- HFE-associated hereditary hemochromatosis is relatively common, affecting 1 in every 250 Caucasian persons in the United States.
- Males are affected by HHC more frequently than females.
- The HFE mutation responsible for type 1 HHC results in increased iron absorption and is characterized by increased iron storage in body tissues such as the liver, pancreas, skin, and heart.
- Hemochromatosis frequently presents with nonspecific symptoms such as abdominal pain, fatigue, and arthralgias.

- Factors that raise clinical suspicion for advanced-stage iron overload include hepatomegaly, hepatic cirrhosis, hepatocellular carcinoma, diabetes mellitus, cardiomyopadism, hypogonadism, arthritis, and hyperpigmented skin.
- Serum ferritin and transferrin saturation have the greatest sensitivity and specificity as biomarkers for hereditary hemochromatosis.
- Liver biopsy is the "gold standard" for assessing the degree of hepatic fibrosis.
- Persons with hemochromatosis are at increased risk for developing hepatocellular carcinoma.
- Therapeutic phlebotomy is the treatment of choice for iron overload.

## Key Terms

**Acute-phase reactant:** any substance that can be elevated in inflammatory processes.

**Alpha-fetoprotein (AFP):** a protein product normally produced only in the fetal liver and used as a tumor marker in adults.

**Aplastic anemia:** a total bone marrow failure characterized by a decrease in all blood cells.

**Cardiomyopathy:** a disease of the myocardium (heart muscle) that has variable etiologies and clinical presentations.

**Carrier:** a term used to describe heterozygotes in recessive disorders who do not express disease characteristics themselves but can pass the mutation on to their offspring.

**Cirrhosis:** a degenerative disease of the liver characterized by formation of fibrous tissue and scarring, resulting in the inhibition of normal cellular function.

**Hepatic ultrasound:** an imaging study of the liver used to detect the presence of tissue changes such as tumors, abscesses, and cysts.

**Hepatitis:** inflammation of the liver causing impaired function as a result of toxins (e.g., alcohol, iron, drugs), autoimmune disorders, or infectious agents (viruses).

**Hepatoma:** the most common type of non-metastatic liver cancer; also known as primary hepatocellular carcinoma.

**Hepatomegaly:** enlargement of the liver.

**Hereditary hemochromatosis:** an autosomal recessive disorder caused by a single mutation in the HFE gene, which causes increased intestinal absorption of iron and results in increased iron storage in body tissues

**Myelodysplastic syndrome:** the underproduction of a single type of blood cell produced in the bone marrow.

**Penetrance:** the proportion of individuals carrying a particular mutation who express an associated, observable trait.

**Point mutation:** the alteration of a single nucleotide to a different nucleotide.

**Polymerase chain reaction (PCR):** repeated cycles of DNA denaturation, renaturation with primer oligonucleotide sequences, and replication, resulting in exponential growth in the number of copies of the DNA sequence located between the primers.

**Serum ferritin levels:** a measure of the amount of iron bound to transferrin.

**Serum iron levels:** a measure of the amount of unbound iron that has been transported to the blood.

**Sex-influenced phenotype:** a phenotype expressed in both male and females but with different frequencies in the two sexes.

**Synergistic hepatotoxic effects:** toxic effects that work together such that the total toxic effect is greater than the sum of the two (or more) single effects.

**Therapeutic phlebotomy:** removal of a portion of the blood volume to alleviate symptoms.

**Total iron-binding capacity (TIBC):** a measure of all proteins available to bind iron and an indirect measure of transferrin levels.

**Transferrin:** the globulin protein that transports iron to the bone marrow.

**Transferrin saturation levels:** the portion of transferrin bound to iron. This value is found by dividing the serum iron by the total iron binding capacity.

**Variable expressivity:** variation in disease symptoms among persons with the same mutation.

## Chapter Review Questions

1. Most hereditary hemochromatosis (HHC) is associated with an HFE mutation and is inherited in a _____ pattern with a disease incidence of _____ in the United States.

2. Early HFE-HHC often manifests clinically with _____, _____, _____, and _____.

3. Serological evidence of iron overload includes elevated _____ and _____.

4. Physical manifestations of iron overload in HFE-HHC include _____, _____, _____, _____, _____, _____, _____, and _____.

5. _____ is the "gold standard" for assessing the presence and amount of hepatic fibrosis.

## Resources

Acton, RT, Barton JC, Adams PC, Speechly MR, et al. Relationship of Serum Ferritin, Transferring Saturation, and HFE Mutations and Self-reported Diabetes in the Hemochromatosis and Iron Overload Screening (HEIRS) Study. *Diabetes Care.* 29(9):2084–2089; 2006.

Adams PC, Reboussin DM, Barton JC, McLaren CR, et al. Hemochromatosis and Iron-Overload Screening in a Racially Diverse Population. *New England Journal of Medicine.* 352:1769–1778; 2005.

Brandhagen DJ, Fairbanks VF, Baldus W. Recognition and Management of Hereditary Hemochromatosis. *American Family Physician.* 65(5):853–860; 2002.

Gene Reviews. www.genetests.org.

Genetics Home Reference. http://ghr.nlm.nih.gov/.

Imperatore G, Pinsky LE, Motulsky A, Reyes M. Hereditary Hemochromatosis: Perspectives of Public Health, Medical Genetics, and Primary Care. *Genetics in Medicine.* 5(1):1–8; 2003.

Morrison ED, Brandhagen DJ, Phatak PD, Barton JC, et al. Serum Ferritin Level Predicts Advanced Hepatic Fibrosis Among U.S. Patients with Phenotypic Hemochromatosis. *Annals of Internal Medicine.* 138:627–633; 2003.

Schmitt B, Golub RM, Green R. Screening Primary Care Patients for Hereditary Hemochromatosis with Transferrin Saturation and Serum Ferritin Level: Systematic Review for the American College of Physicians. *Annals of Internal Medicine.* 143:522–536; 2005.*Stedman's Online Medical Dictionary.* www.stedmans.com.

Tietz NW. *Clinical Guide to Laboratory Tests,* 3rd ed. Philadelphia: W. B. Saunders; 1995.

# Chapter 11

# Cystic Fibrosis

## CHAPTER OBJECTIVES

✓ Describe the etiology and various forms of cystic fibrosis.
✓ Describe related disorders such as congenital absence of vas deferens.
✓ Detail phenotypic features, symptoms, and physical examination findings associated with cystic fibrosis.
✓ Discuss variable expressivity, environmental modifiers, and genetic modifiers.
✓ Review current surveillance and treatment recommendations for cystic fibrosis.

Cystic fibrosis (CF) is a disorder that affects epithelial cells in multiple organ systems. While the most common cause of morbidity associated with CF is pulmonary disease, dysfunction of the exocrine pancreas, intestines, male genitourinary tract, hepatobiliary system, and exocrine glands are also common features of this disease. A mutation in the cystic fibrosis transmembrane conductance regulator (CFTR) gene has been shown to cause this disease.

Inheritance of CF follows an autosomal recessive pattern; thus two copies of the mutated gene are required to cause disease. Among Caucasians in the United States, CF is the most common lethal inherited disorder. The disease incidence is 1 in 3200 live births; the frequency of carriers in the U.S. population is approximately 1 in 25. Cystic fibrosis is more common in persons of Northern European descent and occurs in lower frequencies among other ethnic populations.

## Phenotypic Features

Cystic fibrosis is most commonly a diagnosis made in early childhood, usually during the first year of life. In approximately 5% of cases, patients who are mildly symptomatic are initially diagnosed as adults. Failure to thrive or poor growth rate is a common finding in children. It may be due to malabsorption associated with pancreatic insufficiency, increased caloric expenditure secondary to chronic infection, or both.

Chronic pulmonary infections occur in the majority of patients with CF. The inability of the pulmonary system to mount a defense against pathogens leads to sinusitis in the upper airways and bronchitis in the bronchial tree. The most commonly isolated pathogens in chronic sinus infection and pneumonia are *Staphylococcus aureus* and *Pseudomonas aeruginosa*. Concomitant fungal infections with *Aspergillus fumigates* occur in approximately 10% of CF patients. In the upper airways of persons with CF, nasal polyps, nosebleeds, and chronic sinus infections that are resistant to first-line antibiotics are common.

In the lower airways of CF patients, thick mucus production and neutrophilic inflammation build up to cause airway obstruction. Clinically, this process manifests as a chronic cough with or without sputum production and dyspnea on exertion. After the acute illness subsides, chronic bronchitis persists due to structural changes that have occurred in the airway. Eventually, the functional lung parenchyma is replaced with nonfunctional tissues such as cysts, abscesses, and fibrosis. This effect increases alveolar resistance and results in high blood pressure in the pulmonary artery and the right side of the heart. A sustained high pressure will eventually lead to right-sided heart failure, known as **cor pulmonale**.

Hemoptysis (coughing up blood) is a common presenting feature of CF during periods of acute infection. The chronic inflammation, structural changes, and increased pressure associated with this disease all contribute to damage in the vascular beds. Either chronic blood loss or multiple episodes of massive hemoptysis can result in iron-deficiency anemia in these patients, whereas patients who retain mucus, especially in the upper lobes, may show hyperinflation on chest x-ray.

Pancreatic involvement and gastrointestinal malabsorption are also commonly associated with CF. The pancreas is affected when thickened secretions obstruct the pancreatic ducts, which can lead to inflammation and pancreatitis. Some patients will maintain sufficient pancreatic function with mild inflammation, whereas others will lose pancreatic function. Chronic obstruction of the pancreatic ducts may eventually cause the pancreatic tissues to become fibrotic, resulting in pancreatic insufficiency and decreased or absent digestive enzyme (e.g., amylase, lipase) production. Clinically, this phenomenon is manifested as dietary fats being excreted in the stool (**steatorrhea**) rather than being digested and absorbed. The inability to digest or absorb nutrients, in turn, leads to a decline in growth rate, disorders of blood coagulation, skin rashes, and anemia. Pancreatic insufficiency and malabsorption may be the only symptoms associated with CF in some patients. Approximately 10% of patients with pancreatic insufficiency do not develop pulmonary disease.

While the exocrine pancreas is most often affected by CF-related changes, the endocrine pancreas may also become involved. Both insulin secretion and the number of islet cells are reduced when pancreatic fibrosis occurs. In addition, peripheral insulin resistance has been observed in some patients. When this condition occurs, it is referred to as **cystic fibrosis–related diabetes mellitus**. Although it may present as early as adolescence, its incidence is typically increased in adulthood.

Hepatobiliary disease has a similar pathology to pancreatic disease in patients with CF, in that obstruction of the biliary tract due to thickened mucus can lead to congestion of the liver or **biliary cirrhosis**. As damage to the liver progresses, the patient may experience **portal hypertension** and develop **varices**. Liver disease is the second-leading cause of mortality (after pulmonary disease) in patients with CF.

**Meconium ileus** affects approximately 20% of newborns with CF. This type of intestinal obstruction (ileus) is caused by the presence of unusually thick fetal waste products (meconium). Under normal circumstances, pancreatic enzymes such as trypsin are able to break down the meconium, allowing it to be passed in the feces of the newborn. In the absence of this enzymatic activity (characteristic of CF), the dense meconium is retained in the intestines.

Almost all CF-affected males are infertile due to the absence of spermatozoa (**azoospermia**), which results from the congenital absence of the vas deferens or other supportive structures. Congenital absence of the vas deferens can also occur as the only feature of a CFTR mutation in men without pulmonary or gastrointestinal symptoms. Females with CF are generally ovulatory, but may experience difficulty becoming pregnant if they have abnormal cervical mucus.

Overall, there is a wide variation among affected individuals in terms of the constellation of symptoms, age at presentation, organ system manifestation, severity, and progression of CF. As a result, CF may initially be misdiagnosed as celiac disease, pancreatitis, asthma, or chronic bronchitis. Physical findings are not consistent among affected family members, but rather depend on the severity of CFTR mutations, modifier genes, and environmental factors.

## Genetics

The CFTR gene is the only known gene associated with CF; to date, more than 1000 different mutations in this gene have been identified. Normally, this gene carries instructions for an integral membrane protein that regulates chloride channels in epithelial cells. Under normal physiological conditions, chloride is excreted and excess sodium uptake is inhibited. This process maintains the appropriate water balance in secretions. In CFTR mutations, however, this process is disrupted. In the lungs, this disruption causes defective chloride transport across the membrane (the primary defect) and enhanced sodium absorption (the secondary defect). These changes in ion transport lead to a net increase in water absorption, thinning of the airway surface liquid, and decreased ciliary clearance. In turn, the ability of bacteria to adhere to airway surfaces, proliferate, and resist phagocytosis is enhanced by these changes.

Deletions, nonsense mutations, frameshift mutations, and splice site mutations of the CFTR gene result in the complete absence of a functional CFTR and represent the majority of CF mutations. However, missense mutations appear to only partially alter the function of CFTR. Instead, the amount of functional CFTR seems to determine the clinical presentation and course of disease (**Table 11-1**). Missense mutations often present later in life and may be associated with a milder disease course. It is this variety of mutations in the CFTR gene that is responsible for the variable clinical phenotypes.

The CFTR mutations leading to CF also vary widely among affected kindred and are often scattered across the gene (genetic heterogeneity). Mutations can result in qualitative defects (affecting protein function) or quantitative defects (affecting the amount of functional protein present) of the protein. Within families, variable expressivity of the symptoms is observed. Some affected individuals have multiple or severe symptoms, whereas others exhibit fewer or milder symptoms. It is important to note that the degree of severity in one affected individual does not dictate the degree of severity in that individual's offspring.

Table 11-1 **Relationship Between the Amount of Functional Cystic Fibrosis Transmembrane Conductance Regulator (CFTR) Gene Produced and Phenotypic Expression from CFTR Mutations**

| Percentage of Normal CFTR Function | Manifestations of Cystic Fibrosis |
|---|---|
| < 1% | Classic disease |
| < 4.5% | Progressive pulmonary disease |
| < 5% | Clinically demonstrable sweat abnormality |
| < 10% | Congenital absence of the vas deferens (male infertility) |
| 10–49% | No known abnormality |
| 50–100% | No known abnormality (asymptomatic carriers) |

*Source:* Adapted from www.cysticfibrosismedicine.com.

Cystic fibrosis is inherited in an autosomal recessive pattern. For Caucasians without a family history of CF, the risk of being a carrier of a CFTR mutation is 1 in 25. The risk of a couple having a child with the disease is approximately 1 in 2500. For couples who have one child affected by CF, the risk of CF appearing in future offspring is 1 in 4. Therefore, the risk of inheriting the CFTR mutation in two alleles and developing the disease is 25% if both parents are carriers.

## Diagnosis

The diagnosis of CF may be established in individuals with at least one phenotypic feature and a mutation in CFTR as evidenced by one of the following: (1) presence of two mutations in the CFTR gene; (2) two abnormal quantitative sweat chloride tests (by the quantitative pilocarpine iontophoresis method); or (3) two transepithelial nasal potential difference measurements. The detection rate for CFTR mutations varies depending on the test method employed and the ethnicity of the patient. The quantitative pilocarpine iontophoresis for sweat chloride (commonly referred to as sweat chloride test) is considered the primary test for the diagnosis of CF. This assay reportedly has an accuracy of 90%. Molecular genetic testing is indicated when confirming a positive sweat chloride test, when sweat chloride testing is inconclusive, or when sweat chloride testing is not available. In the rare instance that both sweat chloride testing and mutation testing are either not available or inconclusive; transepithelial nasal potential difference measurements may be used to diagnose CF.

In some special circumstances, the molecular testing method may be used as the first diagnostic study. For example, this technique may be employed for prenatal testing in a high-risk pregnancy, diagnosis in fetuses demonstrating an echogenic bowel on ultrasound, and assessment of symptomatic newborns or other individuals who do not produce adequate volumes of sweat. It is also indicated as the initial test for siblings of an affected proband.

Diagnosis of CF can be made even without phenotypic expression by using newborn screenings and prenatal testing of the amniotic fluid. CFTR mutation testing can be performed using the blood of newborns as well as amniotic fluid taken from their mothers. Sweat chloride testing and transepithelial nasal potential difference are also appropriate screening tests for newborns. In many cases, newborn screening is performed using the immunoreactive trypsinogen assay, which is part of a screening panel routinely applied to blood specimens shortly after birth.

## Genetic Testing and Counseling

Because all CFTR mutations are inherited in an autosomal recessive pattern, the siblings of an affected proband have a 1 in 4 chance of being affected by CF disease and a 1 in 2 chance of being a carrier of a CF-related mutation. Carriers are generally asymptomatic. Most affected individuals with two mutated alleles become symptomatic early in life, so very few parents are initially tested and diagnosed as a result of positive newborn screening. The American College of Medical Geneticists recommends that carrier screening for CF be offered to all Caucasians of non-Jewish descent and Ashkenazi Jews. This assessment is accomplished using a panel of 23 different known mutations that occur in high frequencies among the U.S. population.

## Management, Treatment, and Surveillance

Increased overall survival and enhanced quality of life can be best achieved for those affected with CF when a comprehensive treatment plan is developed after early diagnosis. This plan should include replacement of pancreatic enzymes and deficient vitamins by dietary supplementation, use of bronchodilators to maintain patent airways, antibiotics for respiratory infections, administration of mucus-thinning agents, pain management, anti-inflammatory agents such as ibuprofen, respiratory therapy, and even lung transplant. Attention should be focused on treating disease manifestations as well as preventing future complications.

Treatment of disease manifestations often addresses pulmonary complications by using antibiotics, anti-inflammatory agents, inhaled bronchodilators, mucolytic agents, and chest physiotherapy. Lung transplant may be possible in some patients. Sinus-related complications can be treated using anti-inflammatory agents, antibiotics, and surgical interventions. Chest physiotherapy involves external manual percussion of the chest wall, handheld devices that percuss the chest wall, or inflatable vests that vibrate the chest wall. All of these modalities function to move mucus in the lungs and physically clear obstructed airways. They are usually performed at least twice a day. Collectively, these treatments optimize pulmonary function by opening airways, thinning sputum, allowing secretions to be expectorated, and treating inflammatory and infectious components in as much of the pulmonary surface area as possible.

Immunizations for common pulmonary pathogens are also indicated as preventive measures, including pertussis, measles, varicella, *Haemophilus influenzae* type B, *Streptococcus pneumonia*, respiratory syncytial virus, and influenza virus. Regularly scheduled physical examinations that include pulmonary function testing, chest x-rays, and sputum cultures are important components of pulmonary surveillance. All respiratory irritants—such as smoke, dust, and fumes—should be avoided.

Gastrointestinal complications require nutritional support and enzyme replacement therapy. Indeed, maintaining good growth rates and body weight is crucial to overall health. Patients with a low body mass index (BMI) may benefit from increased caloric intake and use of high-fat supplements under the supervision of a nutritionist specializing in CF. Pancreatic insufficiency can result in low serum protein levels and secondary edema. Pancreatic enzyme and fat-soluble vitamin supplementation are mainstays of prevention. Annual screening of blood glucose levels for CF-related diabetes should be performed; if present, this disease should be managed by an endocrinologist.

Biliary cirrhosis should be suspected when hepatic enzymes (i.e., alanine transaminase [ALT], aspartate transferase [AST]) are elevated. Obstruction of the bile duct can be managed through use of oral bile acids, which dissolve and prevent gallstones. Baseline bone density should be determined in adolescence or as early as possible and repeated annually to detect evolving osteoporosis. Maintaining overall hydration status is also important, as decreased total body water can exacerbate thickening of secretions and associated complications. Regular physical exercise has also been shown to improve bone health and patency of airways.

There is no cure for CF at present. For now, delaying respiratory tract infections and earlier lung transplantation are the most promising therapies. Newer therapies currently under investigation involve methods to bypass CFTR in the ion transport process and improve CFTR protein function.

The improved survival of women with CF is responsible for an increase in the pregnancy rates among these patients. Women with CF should receive prenatal counseling, and should be managed by a team of professionals including a CF specialist, a dietician, and a high-risk obstetrician.

## Associated Syndromes

Males without pulmonary or gastrointestinal manifestations of CF may have congenital absence of the vas deferens (CAVD), a condition that is commonly identified during evaluation for infertility. The diagnosis of CFTR-related CAVD may be established in males with low semen volume, low sperm count, absent or malformed vas deferens on physical examination or imaging, and at least one CFTR mutation. Typically, those affected with CFTR-related CAVD produce semen that has a volume less than 2 mL (normal: 3 – 5 mL), pH < 7.0 (normal > 8.0), elevated citric acid concentration, elevated acid phosphatase concentration, low fructose concentration, and failure to coagulate. A low sperm count (less than 5 million sperm per milliliter of semen) may be a separate indicator or occur in conjunction with low semen volume.

Evidence of structural abnormalities of the seminal vesicles or vas deferens is typically first discovered on physical examination and confirmed by ultrasound imaging. These abnormalities occur in bilateral and unilateral patterns. Testicular function including spermatogenesis is typically normal. Clinical evaluation by a urologist is warranted in any of these circumstances, and disease etiology should be determined by molecular genetic testing for CFTR mutations.

## Chapter Summary

- Cystic fibrosis involves an ion transport disorder in the epithelial cells of multiple organ systems and results in pulmonary disease, pancreatic dysfunction, hepato-biliary disorders, and exocrine dysfunction.

- Cystic fibrosis typically presents in infancy and early childhood.

- The diagnosis of cystic fibrosis is made using screening methods and specific mutation testing.

- Mortality in cystic fibrosis is generally related to pulmonary failure (e.g., pneumonia).

- Surveillance guidelines include population screening.

- Congenital absence of the vas deferens is a disorder related to mutation in the CFTR gene.

## Key Terms

**Azoospermia:** the absence of spermatozoa in the semen.

**Biliary cirrhosis:** cirrhosis due to biliary obstruction, which may be a primary intrahepatic disease or occur secondary to obstruction of extrahepatic bile ducts.

**Cor pulmonale:** failure of the right ventricle of the heart, secondary to enlargement and increased pressure caused by disease of the lungs or pulmonary blood vessels.

**Cystic fibrosis–related diabetes mellitus:** insulin deficiency and insulin resistance caused by complications from cystic fibrosis.

**Meconium ileus:** obstruction of the intestines due to retention of a dark green waste product (meconium) that is normally passed shortly after a child's birth.

**Portal hypertension:** elevation of pressure in the hepatic portal circulation due to cirrhosis or other fibrotic change in liver tissue. When pressure exceeds 10 mm Hg, a collateral circulation may develop to maintain venous return from structures drained by the portal vein; engorgement of collateral veins can lead to esophageal varices and, less often, caput medusae.

**Steatorrhea:** excretion of excess fat in the feces.

**Varices:** an enlarged and tortuous vein, artery, or lymphatic vessel.

## Chapter Review Questions

1. Cystic fibrosis is the result of a mutation in the _____ gene.

2. The most life-threatening complication associated with cystic fibrosis is _____.

3. The chance of two carriers having offspring with cystic fibrosis is_____, which is described as an _____ pattern of inheritance.

4. Physical examination findings that raise clinical suspicion for cystic fibrosis in infants and young children include _____, _____, and _____.

5. Infertile males without pulmonary or gastrointestinal manifestations of cystic fibrosis may have _____.

## Resources

Anson DS, Smith GJ, Parsons DW. Gene Therapy for Cystic Fibrosis Airway Disease. *Current Gene Therapy.* 6:161–179; 2006.

Bennett C, Peckham D. The Genetics of Cystic Fibrosis [online]. Leeds, UK: Leeds University Teaching Hospitals; August 2002. http://www.cysticfibrosismedicine .com.

Cystic Fibrosis Foundation. www.cff.rog.

Cystic Fibrosis Medicine. http://www.cysticfibrosismedicine.com. Gene Reviews. www .ncbi.nlm.nih.

Goss CH, Newsom SA, Schildcrout JS, Sheppard L, et al. Effect of Ambient Air Pollution on Pulmonary Exacerbations and Lung Function in Cystic Fibrosis. *American Journal Respiratory Critical Care Medicine.* 169:816–821; 2004.

Moskowitz SM, Chmiel JF, Sternen DL, Cheng E, et al. Clinical Practice and Genetic Counseling for Cystic Fibrosis and CFTR-Related Disorders. *Genetics in Medicine.* 10(12):851–868; 2008.

Nick JA, Rodman DM. Manifestations of Cystic Fibrosis Diagnosed in Adulthood. *Current Opinion in Pulmonary Medicine.* 11:513–518; 2005.

Vanscoy LL, Blackman SM, Collaco JM, Bowers A, et al. Heritability of Lung Disease Severity in Cystic Fibrosis. *American Journal Respiratory Critical Care Medicine.* 175: 1036–1043; 2007.

# Chapter 12

# Familial Thoracic Aortic Aneurysms and Dissections

## CHAPTER OBJECTIVES

✓ Describe the etiology and various forms of familial thoracic aortic aneurysms and dissections.

✓ Detail symptoms associated with familial thoracic aortic aneurysms and dissections.

✓ Discuss penetrance and variable expressivity.

✓ Review other syndromes associated with familial thoracic aneurysms and dissections.

✓ Review current surveillance and treatment recommendations for familial thoracic aneurysms and dissections.

A **thoracic aortic aneurysm** is widening or bulging of the upper portion of the aorta that may occur in the descending thoracic aorta, the ascending aorta, or the aortic arch. **Aortic dissection** is a longitudinal tear between the layers of the aorta that may progress due to the high-pressure flow inside the aorta. Familial thoracic aortic aneurysm and dissection (TAAD) is a confirmed diagnosis of thoracic aortic aneurysm in any individual with a positive family history of thoracic aortic aneurysm. This disorder is the thirteenth-leading cause of death in the United States, accounting for nearly 15,000 deaths annually. Approximately 20% of thoracic aortic aneurysms and dissections result from a familial predisposition.

The aorta is the largest artery in the body. Like all arteries, it is composed of three different layers. The innermost layer in direct contact with blood is the intima; it is composed of endothelial cells. The middle layer, the media, is made up of smooth muscle cells and elastic tissue. The outermost layer of connective tissue is known as the adventitia.

In aortic dissection, the tear begins in the intima and progresses to the media. The increased pressure associated with this blood flow damages and tears the media, allowing more blood to fill and divide the layers. This division continues along the length of aorta toward the heart, away from the heart, or in both directions. The onset and rate of progression of the aortic dilatation vary among affected persons. However, if this condition is not identified and treated, the aorta may eventually rupture and lead to a massive hemorrhage that usually proves fatal. Unfortunately, aortic dissection is a medical emergency that can lead to sudden death, even with appropriate treatment.

## Diagnosis

Familial thoracic aortic aneurysm and dissection is diagnosed based on the presence of dilation and/or dissection of the thoracic aorta and a positive family history that is not attributable to **Marfan syndrome** or other connective tissue abnormalities. The major diagnostic criteria for TAAD include the presence of dilatation and/or dissection of the ascending thoracic aorta or dissection of the descending aorta distal to the subclavian artery. Diagnosis is confirmed by measuring the dimensions of the aorta at the level of the sinuses of Valsalva and by measuring the ascending aorta using either computerized tomography (CT), magnetic resonance imaging (MRI), or trans-esophageal echocardiography. These dimensions are then compared to age-appropriate nomograms that have been adjusted for body surface area. The progressive enlargement of the ascending aorta can involve sinuses of Valsalva, ascending aorta, or both. When making a diagnosis of TAAD, it is also necessary to specifically exclude Marfan syndrome, Loeys-Deitz syndrome, and other connective tissue abnormalities. Both family history and genetic testing are helpful in this regard.

While plain films (x-rays) are not the diagnostic imaging study of choice for TAAD, posterior–anterior and lateral views of the chest are often the first imaging studies ordered for the patient presenting with a chief complaint of "chest pain." Abnormal chest x-ray findings that should raise suspicion of TAAD include an enlarged aortic knob or localized bulge, widened mediastinum, extension of the aortic shadow beyond a calcified wall, and longitudinal aortic enlargement. A double density of the aorta may also be evident because the false lumen is less radiopaque than the true lumen. The loss of space between the aorta and the pulmonic artery (the aortopulmonic window) on the posterior–anterior view is also indicative of aneurysm or dissection.

Plain films of the chest are not diagnostically reliable for aortic dissection, however, and TAAD may not be excluded based on a normal chest x-ray. Echocardiography, CT, and MRI are imaging modalities that are useful in the diagnosis of TAAD and should be considered even in the absence of findings on plain films. Recent changes in the recommendations for persons with a family history of TAAD require that all first-degree relatives of the affected proband have an initial screening to measure the aortic root diameter and follow-up imaging to evaluate disease progression at regular intervals.

For an initial screening, CT is generally preferred for several reasons. For example, CT is more readily available, is noninvasive, and is more easily tolerated by the patient. MRI is often contraindicated in patients requiring aortic imaging, such as in persons with implanted pacemakers or other metallic devices. Both MRI and CT measure the external aortic diameter, making either modality preferred over echocardiogram. However, the CT measures from the center of intraluminal flow to each side of the aortic wall, giving a more accurate representation of the true diameter. For acute dissection, CT is also a more rapid diagnostic tool. Regardless of which imaging modality is used, providers should consider specific elements when evaluating reports of TAAD to include location of measurements, filling defects, presence of genetic syndromes, and comparison of any prior images.

**Table 12-1   Aortic Dissection Bundle Questions to Assess Risk of Familial Thoracic Aortic Aneurysm and Dissection**

Does the patient's family have a history of aortic dissection?

Does the patient have Marfan syndrome or a family history of Marfan syndrome?

Do physical findings suggest the patient may have undiagnosed Marfan syndrome?

Note: A single "yes" answer means that aortic dissection may be the cause of the patient's pain, and the diagnosis should be excluded by emergent computerized tomography scan, magnetic resonance imaging, or transesophageal echocardiogram.

*Source:* Adapted from Best Care News. Methodist Health System. Available at http://www.bestcare .org/mhsbase/mhs.cfm/SRC=MD010/SRCN=newsdetail/GnavID=71/ HLNewsItemID=239. Accessed January 20, 2010.

When screening patients of any age for the chief complaint of "chest pain," it is strongly suggested that the aortic dissection bundle questions be included in the initial patient history (**Table 12-1**). These questions can help identify patients at risk for TAAD based on personal and family history by prompting the clinician to include TAAD in the differential diagnosis for chest pain. Electrocardiogram (ECG) findings may be normal or show nonspecific changes such as left ventricular hypertrophy or blocks. If the patient has previously undergone ECG, it may be helpful to compare new findings with baseline studies. Sinus tachycardia is the most common abnormal ECG finding.

The primary manifestation of TAAD may be (1) dilatation of the aorta at the level of the ascending aorta or at the level of the sinuses of Valsalva, (2) dissection of the ascending aorta, or (3) both. Affected individuals typically have progressive enlargement of the ascending aorta leading to either an aortic dissection involving the ascending aorta (type A dissection) or rupture (**Figure 12-1**). Dissections may also begin in the arch or distal to the arch and propagate distally (type B dissection).

Clinical features of aortic aneurysms and dissection includes severe pain in the anterior chest, posterior chest, or both. Pain may also be referred to either shoulder, but is most commonly noted in the left shoulder. When the tear involves the abdominal aorta, abdominal pain may be the predominant feature. Dissections can also cause other signs and symptoms including "the four Ps": pallor, pulselessness, paresthesias, and paralysis. When blood fills the dissection, it is not available in the general circulation, resulting in loss of perfusion to extremities and vital organs. This shunting can contribute to pulse deficits—a major physical examination finding in TAAD. Paresthesias are another manifestation of decreased peripheral perfusion. Paralysis results from nerve compression by the enlarging aneurysmal sac. This constellation of signs and symptoms is frequently misdiagnosed as a cerebrovascular accident or "stroke." Younger persons presenting with TAAD are most likely to be misdiagnosed with pulmonary causes of chest pain such as pleurisy, bronchitis, or pneumonia.

In families with TAAD, one individual in the family may present with an **aortic aneurysm** at a young age, whereas another individual may present at an elderly age—a phenomenon

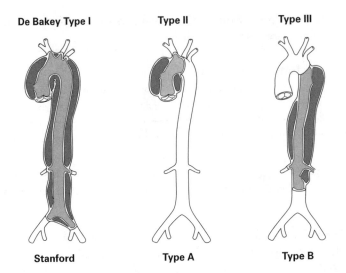

**De Bakey**

Type I: Originates in the ascending aorta, propagates at least to the aortic arch, and often beyond it distally.

Type II: Originates in and is confined to the ascending aorta.

Type III: Originates in the descending aorta and extends distally down the aorta or, rarely, retrograde into the aortic arch and ascending aorta.

**Stanford**

Type A: All dissections involving the ascending aorta, regardless of the site of origin.

Type B: All dissections not involving the ascending aorta.

**Figure 12-1** Stanford and DeBakey classification systems for thoracic aortic dissection.
*Source:* Nienaber CA, Eagle KA. Aortic Dissection: New Frontiers in Diagnosis and Management: Part I: From Etiology to Diagnostic Strategies. *Circulation.* 108:628–635; 2003.

known as **variable expressivity**. Notably, the mean age of presentation of individuals with familial TAAD is younger than that of individuals with nonfamilial TAAD, but generally older than the mean age of presentation of individuals who have Marfan syndrome. Aortic dissection is exceedingly rare in persons younger than the age of 16, but aortic dilatation may be present in childhood.

Members of some families with TAAD have been observed to have an increase in inguinal hernias and scoliosis. The propensity for arterial dilatation results in aneurysms in other locations along the aorta as well as cerebral aneurysms. A minority of these families have an increased incidence of bicuspid aortic valve.

The pathological basis for weakening of the aortic wall in familial TAAD is cystic medial necrosis. In this process, the middle layer (media) of the aorta loses smooth muscle fibers and hence elasticity. These cells are replaced with mucoid material, which is less elastic and weakens the walls of the aorta.

# Genetic Testing and Counseling

Four genes—*TGFBR2, TGFBR1, MYH11, and ACTA2*—found at either of two loci (FAA1 and TAAD1) are known to be associated with TAAD. Molecular genetic testing for all four associated genes at these two loci is available.

TAAD1 mutations and *ACTA2* mutations account for the majority of mutations in TAAD families, and all mutations appear to be inherited in an autosomal dominant manner. The majority of those individuals who are diagnosed with TAAD also have an affected parent. Siblings of the proband are at increased risk depending on the status of the parents. For this reason, it is important to evaluate both parents and all siblings of those individuals positively or presumptively diagnosed with TAAD. Parents, siblings, and offspring of a proband have a 50% risk of having TAAD.

Affected persons with *TGFBR2* mutations may experience aortic dissection at aortic dilatation of 5.0 centimeters, which is well below the average threshold of 6.0 centimeters. These individuals frequently present with aortic disease and have an increased risk for aneurysms and dissection of other vessels such as cerebral arteries.

**Penetrance** is indicated by the proportion of individuals carrying a particular mutation who also express an associated, observable trait. Persons with mutation of the FAA1 gene show full penetrance of aortic dilation and dissection, whereas individuals with TAAD1 mutations show decreased penetrance (especially among women). Mutations in *MYH11* have been associated with patent ductus arteriosus. **Livedo reticularis** and **iris flocculi** are physical findings associated with families demonstrating mutations of the *ACTA2* gene. Iris flocculi are an ocular abnormality found in persons with familial TAAD (**Figure 12-2**). Livedo

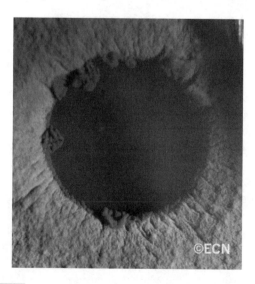

**Figure 12-2** Iris flocculi at the pupillary margin as observed by high-powered slit lamp.
*Source:* Courtesy of Dr. Paul Finger. http://www.eyecancer.com.

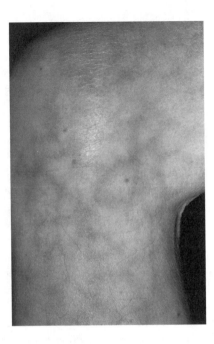

**Figure 12-3** Example of livedo reticularis.
*Source:* Dr. P. Marazzi/Photo Researchers, Inc.

reticularis manifests as a purplish skin discoloration in a lacy pattern caused by constriction of deep dermal capillaries (**Figure 12-3**).

## Management and Treatment

Initial evaluations that are recommended for TAAD include echocardiography of the aorta and aortic valve and cerebrovascular imaging to identify any other aneurysms. Physical examination for inguinal hernias and scoliosis should be performed with appropriate follow-up testing for any abnormal findings. Ocular examination to exclude lens displacement (ectopia lentis) due to Marfan syndrome is also indicated.

Control of hypertension is essential in managing TAAD. For example, beta-adrenergic blocking agents are commonly used to reduce hemodynamic stress when aortic dilatation is present. Surgical repair of asymptomatic thoracic aortic aneurysms is indicated to prevent future dissection or rupture. Criteria for prophylactic repair include dilation that increases at a rate of 1.0 centimeter annually or the presence of aortic regurgitation. For TAAD associated with *TGFBR2* mutations and in persons with a bicuspid aortic valve, the threshold undertaking for such repair is reached when the ascending aorta is 5.0 centimeters in diameter. For other individuals, the threshold for prophylactic repair is an ascending aortic diameter of 5.0 to 5.5 centimeters. Any individuals with a family history of dissection or rupture without prior evidence of aortic root enlargement should undergo earlier repair.

Just as in Marfan syndrome, pregnancy represents a special circumstance for women with TAAD. During pregnancy, labor, delivery, and the postpartum period, the aortic root may enlarge at an increased rate due to the changing hemodynamics associated with pregnancy. Dissection and rupture are more common during this time, so close monitoring of these patients is recommended. Women with TAAD should receive care from a high-risk obstetrician and a cardiologist during their pregnancy.

Surveillance measures for stable individuals should include annual examinations and echocardiogram to monitor the status of the aorta. More frequent exams and imaging studies are indicated for those persons with larger aortic dimensions or rapid rates of dilatation. Individuals who require closer surveillance include those with an aortic root diameter greater than 4.5 centimeters, those whose aortic growth rate exceeds 0.5 centimeter annually, and those with evidence of aortic regurgitation.

All first-degree relatives of affected individuals should be assessed annually by echocardiogram to evaluate the ascending aorta. It is recommended that the entire aorta be imaged every 4 to 5 years by CT or MRI angiography, with this surveillance beginning at 6 to 7 years of age. All previously undiagnosed individuals who are found to have abnormalities by this screening should have their first-degree relatives screened as well. Furthermore, any sons of women who are first-degree relatives of an affected individual should be screened regardless of the mother's echocardiogram results, because decreased penetrance is common in women. Avoidance of isometric exercises (weight lifting), rapid deceleration (motor vehicle accidents), and contact sports is recommended, as these activities may contribute to accelerated dilatation, dissection, and rupture.

## Associated Syndromes

Marfan syndrome is primarily associated with FBN1 mutations, but may also be seen in conjunction with *TGFBR2* mutations, similar to TAAD. Marfan syndrome is inherited in an autosomal dominant pattern (see Chapter 15).

Loeys-Dietz syndrome is caused by mutations in the *TGFBR1* and *TGFBR2* genes. It is characterized by aneurysms, arterial dissections and tortuosities, craniofacial abnormalities, and skeletal abnormalities. The mode of inheritance for this syndrome is also autosomal dominant.

## Chapter Summary

- Familial thoracic aortic aneurysm and dissection is caused by connective tissue defects that result in a loss of smooth muscle fibers and elasticity, thereby weakening the aorta and other arteries.

- Familial thoracic aortic aneurysm and dissection typically presents at an earlier age than sporadic thoracic aneurysm.

- Familial thoracic aortic aneurysm and dissection is diagnosed based on the presence of dilation and/or dissection of the thoracic aorta and a positive family history that is not attributable to Marfan syndrome or other connective tissue abnormalities.

- The aortic dissection bundle questions should be included in the initial history for all patients complaining of chest pain regardless of age.

- The most common presenting complaint with familial thoracic aortic aneurysm and dissection is ripping or tearing chest pain that may be associated with pallor, pulse deficits, paresthesias, and paralysis.

- Surveillance guidelines for first-degree relatives include annual imaging of the aorta beginning in childhood.

- Pregnancy presents a special surveillance consideration as women with familial thoracic aortic aneurysm and dissection are at increased risk for aortic dissection and rupture.

## Key Terms

**Aortic aneurysm:** an abnormal dilation of the aorta at the level of the ascending aorta or the sinuses of Valsalva (descending aorta).

**Aortic dissection:** a longitudinal tear between the layers of the aorta that may progress due to the high-pressure flow inside the aorta.

**Iris flocculi:** an ocular abnormality found in persons with familial thoracic aortic aneurysms and dissections that is highly associated with *ACTA2* mutations.

**Livedo reticularis:** a purplish skin discoloration in a lacy pattern caused by constriction of deep dermal capillaries.

**Marfan syndrome:** a connective tissue, multisystemic disorder characterized by skeletal changes (arachnodactyly, long limbs, joint laxity), cardiovascular defects (aortic aneurysm that may dissect, mitral valve prolapse), and ectopia lentis. It is passed on through autosomal dominant inheritance of a mutation in the fibrillin-1 gene on chromosome 15.

**Penetrance:** the proportion of individuals carrying a particular mutation who express an associated, observable trait.

**Thoracic aortic aneurysm:** widening or bulging of the upper portion of the aorta that may occur in the descending thoracic aorta, the ascending aorta, or the aortic arch.

**Variable expressivity:** variation in disease symptoms among persons with the same mutation.

## Chapter Review Questions

1. The majority of familial thoracic aortic aneurysms and dissections are the result of mutations in the _____ and _____ genes.

2. The most life-threatening complication associated with thoracic aortic aneurysms and dissections is _____.

3. The chance of an affected individual having offspring with familial thoracic aortic aneurysm and dissection is _____, which is described as an _____ pattern of inheritance.

4. Signs and symptoms that raise clinical suspicion for familial thoracic aortic aneurysms and dissections include _____, _____, _____, and _____.

5. Initial recommended evaluations for familial thoracic aortic aneurysms and dissections include _____ of the aorta and aortic valve and _____ to identify any other aneurysms.

## Resources

Albornoz G, Coady MA, Roberts M, Davies RR, et al. Familial Thoracic Aortic Aneurysm and Dissections: Incidence, Modes of Inheritance, and Phenotypic Patterns. *Annals of Thoracic Surgery.* 82:1400–1406; 2006.

Biddinger A, Rocklin M, Coselli J, Milewicz DM. Familial thoracic Aortic Dilations and Dissections: A Case Control Study. *Journal of Vascular Surgery.* 25:506–511; 1997.

Gene Reviews. www.ncbi.nlm.nih.

Hasham SN, Guo DC, Milewicz DM. Genetic Basis of Thoracic Aortic Aneurysms and Dissections. *Current Opinions in Cardiology.* 17:677–683; 2002.

Hasham SN, Lewin, MR, Tran VT, et al. Nonsyndromic Genetic Predisposition to Aortic Dissection: A Newly Recognized, Diagnosable, and Preventable Occurrence In Families. *Annals of Emergency Medicine.* 43:79–82; 2004.

Hiratzka LF, Bakris GL, Beckman JA, Bersin RM, Carr VF, Casey DE, et al. 2010 ACCF/AHA/AATS/ACR/ASA/SCA/SCAI/SIR/STS/SVM Guidelines for Diagnosis and Management of Patients with Thoracic Aortic Disease: Executive Summary. *Circulation.* 121:1544–1579; 2010.

Milewicz DM, Chen H, Park ES, Petty EM, Zaghi H, Shashidhar G, et al. Reduced Penetrance and Variable Expressivity of Familial Thoracic Aortic Aneurysms/ Dissections. *American Journal of Cardiology.* 82:474–479; 1998. [PubMed]

Nienaber CA, Eagle KA. Aortic dissection: New Frontiers in Diagnosis and Management: Part I: From Etiology to Diagnostic Strategies. *Circulation.* 108:628–635; 2003.

Singh KK, Rommel K, Mishra A, Karck M, Haverich A, Schmidtke J, Arslan-Kirchner M. *TGFBR1* and *TGFBR2* Mutations in Patients with Features of Marfan Syndrome and Loeys-Dietz Syndrome. *Human Mutations.* 27:770–777; 2006.

*Stedman's Online Medical Dictionary.* www.stedmans.com.

# Chapter 13

# Familial Hypercholesterolemia

## CHAPTER OBJECTIVES

✓ Describe the etiology and various forms of familial hypercholesterolemia.
✓ Detail symptoms associated with familial hypercholesterolemia.
✓ Discuss allelic variants, loss-of-function mutations, and gain-of-function mutations.
✓ Review current screening and treatment recommendations for familial hypercholesterolemia.

Hypercholesterolemia is defined as a fasting total blood **cholesterol** level of more than 240 mg/dL. While more than 34 million American adults have elevated blood cholesterol levels, the inherited forms of hypercholesterolemia are less common. The most widely inherited form of high cholesterol, called familial hypercholesterolemia (FH), affects approximately 1 in every 500 people. Familial hypercholesterolemia is characterized by increased levels of total serum cholesterol (TC) with increased **low-density lipoprotein** cholesterol (LDL-C), tendinous xanthomata, and premature symptoms of coronary heart disease. This clinical phenotype may be inherited in either an autosomal dominant pattern or an autosomal recessive pattern, depending on the specific mutation. In all cases, the phenotype is associated with premature death. Persons with FH usually have higher levels of TC compared with the general population. A higher frequency of FH is noted to occur among certain populations such as South Africans, French Canadians, Lebanese, and Finns. These populations are responsible for the random genetic mutation that occurs as a result of its proliferation from only a few parent colonizers—a phenomenon known as the **founder effect**.

## Genetics

The low-density lipoprotein receptor (LDLR) protein is encoded on the LDLR gene. This receptor binds to LDL particles that function as carriers for cholesterol in the blood. Under normal circumstances, these receptors function to eliminate LDL from the blood, thereby regulating TC levels. However, in FH, the cell surface receptors for LDL may be defective or absent, resulting in unregulated synthesis of LDL-C. When LDL receptors are absent or have diminished ability to function, excess cholesterol accumulates in the body and is deposited in tissues in abnormal amounts. The skin, tendons, and arteries are the tissues that are most commonly affected by this problem.

When the LDLR gene is absent, the phenotype has even more severe effects compared to the phenotype expressed for LDLR gene defects. To date, more than 1000 different defects, known as **allelic variants**, have been identified in the LDLR gene. When this defect exists in the homozygous state (two affected genes), **atherosclerosis** develops in early childhood and serum cholesterol levels may reach be as much as eight times the upper limits of normal. Affected individuals may require liver transplantation to decrease hepatic lipid production and ameliorate the disease process.

The homozygous form of FH is relatively rare (1 in 1 million) and is detectable at birth. The heterozygous manifestation (only one affected gene) of the disease presents clinically with serum LDL-C levels that are two times the upper limits of normal. Atherosclerotic disease begins to develop in the third and fourth decades of life in these individuals. The incidence of heterozygous FH is approximately 1 in 500, making it roughly 2000 times more common than the homozygous expression.

## Environmental Risk Factors

High blood cholesterol levels in the general population typically result from a combination of genetic and environmental risk factors. Lifestyle choices including diet, exercise, and tobacco smoking strongly influence the amount of cholesterol in the blood. Other factors that affect cholesterol levels include a person's gender, age, and chronic health problems such as diabetes and obesity. The extent to which these environmental risk factors increase morbidity and mortality specific to FH is not known.

## Physical Examination Findings

Cholesterol is a fatty substance that is produced in the liver and can also be obtained from animal-based foods such as eggs, meat, and dairy products. Not all cholesterol is necessarily bad. In fact, cholesterol is an integral part of cellular membranes and certain steroid hormones, and it aids in the digestion of dietary fats. Nevertheless, it has been well documented that high blood cholesterol levels contribute to the development of atherosclerosis and are a risk factor for heart attack and stroke.

When present in excess amounts in the blood, cholesterol is deposited onto the walls of blood vessels such as the coronary arteries that supply blood to the heart. These deposits are known as plaques. Development of atherosclerosis begins with an injury to the endothelium of the vessel wall; inflammation, infection, smoking, and elevated LDL-C, for example, can all cause the initial injury. Once injured, LDL-C enters the vessel wall and the LDL-C particles become oxidized and recruit blood monocytes to the site of injury. The monocytes phagocytize the LDL-C particles, which results in the microscopic appearance of "foamy," lipid-laden macrophages (known as foam cells).

Eventually, as the disease progresses, the heavy burden of lipids in individual cells causes cellular death, leaving behind cholesterol crystals in the plaque. The plaque can either cause obstruction of the lumen of the vessel (occlusion) or rupture. When the vessel is obstructed by 70%, ischemic symptoms may develop, such as **angina**—chest pain that is associated with exercise or physical activity and is relieved by rest. When the plaque ruptures, it becomes a circulating thrombus that may completely occlude smaller vessels, such as the coronary arteries that provide blood to the myocardium. When blood flow is blocked to the distal tissues, cell death—otherwise known as **myocardial infarction** or heart attack—occurs. This permanent damage may be fatal if it is extensive enough to prevent normal cardiac function.

Cholesterol deposits that accumulate in tendons cause abnormal growths known as tendon **xanthomas**. Most commonly, these growths involve the Achilles tendon as well as tendons in the hands and fingers. Similar deposits in the skin result in xanthomas and **xanthelasmata**, which are yellowish cholesterol deposits under the skin or under the eyelids, respectively. Cholesterol may also be deposited at the peripheral border of the cornea, resulting in **arcus corneus**.

## Related Disorders

In addition to the LDLR mutation, mutations in some other genes have also been shown to cause hypercholesterolemia. Mutations in the *APOB*, *LDLRAP1*, and *PCSK9* genes result in increased blood cholesterol and are not uncommon.

Various *APOB* gene mutations result in a type of inherited hypercholesterolemia known as familial defective apolipoprotein B-100. Each of these mutations changes a single amino acid in a critical region of the gene, which inhibits normal binding of LDL-C particles to cell surface receptors. Consequently, fewer LDL-C particles are removed from the blood and circulating cholesterol levels increase (Genetics Home Reference, 2010).

*LDLARP1* mutations are linked to an autosomal recessive inheritance pattern of hypercholesterolemia. A variety of mutations in this gene have been shown to either diminish the amount of protein synthesized or lead to production of an abnormal protein. While the receptors maintain their ability to bind LDL-C particles, they are not able to transport them across the cell membrane, thus allowing the cholesterol particles to accumulate in the blood.

The *PCSK9* gene encodes instructions for the protein that determines the number of LDL receptors. This protein breaks down LDL receptors before they reach the cell surface, thereby controlling cholesterol levels. A **gain-of-function mutation** in *PCSK9* enhances the normal activity of the protein. In this case, there is increased destruction of LDL-C receptors, which in turn results in increased circulating LDL-C levels. Other I gene mutations may result in diminished normal activity. In such a case, more LDL receptors would reach the cell surface and be able to bind more LDL-C, thereby reducing the amount of circulating LDL cholesterol in the blood. Such a mutation leading to decreased normal activity is known as a **loss-of-function mutation**. In any case, hypercholesterolemia results when the LDLRs are unable to effectively remove cholesterol from the blood.

## Environmental and Other Factors

The interaction between genes and environmental factors as demonstrated in FH is unclear. Increased age, obesity, diabetes, lipid levels, and smoking are all strong predictors of risk independent of mutation status. When stratifying risk, modifiable lifestyle changes should be considered in early intervention and prevention strategies.

Factors that may cause an increase in TC include hypothyroidism, nephrotic syndrome, chronic renal insufficiency, liver disease, menopause, and Cushing's disease. In addition, drugs that may increase TC levels include anabolic steroids, oral contraceptives, diuretics, and some α-blockers. It is prudent to rule out secondary causes of abnormal lipid results before initiating lipid-lowering pharmacotherapy.

## Testing

Today, routine screening tools for hypercholesterolemia include family history, pedigree, and a fasting lipid profile. Mutation testing is currently not commonly performed, but its use is projected to grow among families in whom early coronary heart disease is prevalent. Obviously, it is important for the clinician to have an understanding of the most up-to-date cholesterol screening guidelines for various patient populations (**Tables 13-1 and 13-2**). Adults with other coronary risk factors or equivalents such as peripheral artery disease, aortic aneurysm, carotid artery disease, or diabetes should be screened and monitored more closely.

Children and adolescents should be screened selectively for dyslipidemia when they meet one of the following criteria: (1) family history of coronary heart disease, (2) one parent with a TC greater than 240 mg/dL, or (3) one other risk factor such as high blood pressure, smoking, sedentary lifestyle, obesity, alcohol intake, drug use, or presence of disease known to be associated with dyslipidemia (i.e., diabetes). Their risk is stratified using established cholesterol level criteria for children between the ages of 2 to 19 (Table 13-2). Special consideration should also be given to other high-risk populations, such as persons on antiretroviral therapy used in HIV infection, patients with liver disease, and postmenopausal females. As yet, no screening criteria have been established for these populations.

**Table 13-1  Adult (Age Older Than 19) National Cholesterol Education Program Guidelines for Total Cholesterol and Low-Density Lipoprotein Cholesterol**

|  | Acceptable | Borderline | High |
| --- | --- | --- | --- |
| Total cholesterol | < 200 | 200–240 | > 240 |
| LDL cholesterol | < 130 | 130–160 | > 160 |

*Source:* Adapted from the National Heart, Lung, and Blood Institute. Third Report of the Expert Panel on Detection, Evaluation, and Treatment of High Blood Cholesterol in Adults (ATP III Final Report). Available at http://www.nhlbi.nih.gov/guidelines/cholesterol. Accessed January 20, 2010.

Table 13-2  **Child and Adolescent (Ages 2 to 19) National Cholesterol Education Program Guidelines for Total Cholesterol and Low-Density Lipoprotein Cholesterol**

|  | Acceptable | Borderline | High |
|---|---|---|---|
| Total cholesterol | <170 | 170–199 | > 200 |
| LDL cholesterol | < 110 | 110–129 | > 130 |

*Source:* Adapted from the National Heart, Lung, and Blood Institute. Third Report of the Expert Panel on Detection, Evaluation, and Treatment of High Blood Cholesterol in Adults (ATP III Final Report). Available at http://www.nhlbi.nih.gov/guidelines/cholesterol. Accessed January 20, 2010.

Another consideration is how lipids are analyzed and reported by clinical laboratories. For example, TC level alone is not valuable unless fractionated values for high-density lipoprotein cholesterol (HDL-C) and LDL-C are also available. Unlike other parameters, there is no established "reference range" for blood lipids. Instead, risk is stratified by desired levels and is expressed as "acceptable," "borderline," or "high" depending on TC and LDL-C levels (Tables 13-1 and 13-2).

Finally, it is important to understand the relationship of the various lipid fractions to coronary risk. Three different lipoproteins carry cholesterol and are classified based on their density and composition: (1) very-low-density lipoprotein cholesterol (VLDL-C), which is the greatest measure of triglycerides (TG); (2) LDL-C; and (3) HDL-C. The TC measure roughly translate into the sum of these components. The majority of clinical laboratories directly analyze TC, total TG, and the HDL-C, whereas LDL-C levels are calculated using the following equation:

$$LDL\text{-}C = TC - HDL\text{-}C - TG/5$$

The American Heart Association recommends that at least three fasting lipid profiles be performed as baseline testing before initiating lipid-lowering therapy. When hyperlipidemia of any type is confirmed by this method, a phenotype may be determined according to the Fredrickson classification (**Table 13-3**). This classification serves as an aid in selecting appropriate pharmacotherapeutic agents. The family history and pedigree should include identification of kindred with known cardiovascular disease, smoking history, hypertension, age at diagnosis, presence of diabetes or other major illness, gender, longevity, and cause of death (**Table 13-4**).

## Management and Surveillance

The current target goal for LDL-C is less than 100 mg/dL. Pharmacotherapy is beneficial in FH heterozygotes, using either lipid-lowering statins or statin/bile resin combination therapies (**Table 13-5**). Statins remain the most effective agents for lowering LDL-C by inhibition of the enzyme that is responsible for endogenous hepatic cholesterol production—namely, 3-hydroxy-3-methylglutaryl-coenzyme A reductase (HMG-CoA reductase).

**Table 13-3　Lipoprotein Phenotyping (Frederickson Classification) of Lipid Disorders**

| Type | Appearance | Elevated Particles | Associated Clinical Disorders | Serum TC | Serum TG |
|------|-----------|-------------------|------------------------------|----------|----------|
| I | Creamy top | Chylomicrons | Primary to familial lipoprotein lipase deficiency, apolipoprotein C-II deficiency<br>Secondary to uncontrolled diabetes, systemic lupus erythematosus, dysgammaglobulinemia | → | ↓↓ |
| IIa | Clear | LDL | Primary to familial hypercholesterolemia, polygenic hypercholesterolemia, familial combined hyperlipidemia<br>Secondary to nephrotic syndrome, dysgammaglobulinemia, hypothyroidism | ↑↑ | → |
| IIb | Clear | LDL, VLDL | Primary to familial combined hyperlipidemia, familial hypercholesterolemia, hyper-pre-β-lipoproteinemia.<br>Secondary to nephrotic syndrome, dysgammaglobulinemia, hypothyroidism | ↑↑ | ↑ |
| III | Turbid | IDL | Primary to dysbetalipoproteinemia, apolipoprotein E3 deficiency<br>Secondary to uncontrolled diabetes, hypothyroidism, dysgammaglobulinemia, alcohol excess | ↑ | ↑ |

*Continues*

**Table 13-3  Lipoprotein Phenotyping (Frederickson Classification) of Lipid Disorders** (*Continued*)

| Type | Appearance | Elevated Particles | Associated Clinical Disorders | Serum TC | Serum TG |
|------|-----------|--------------------|-------------------------------|----------|----------|
| IV | Turbid | VLDL | Primary to familial hyper-triglyceridemia, familial combined hyperlipidemia, sporadic hypertriglyceridemia<br>Secondary to uncontrolled diabetes, nephrotic syndrome, dysgamma- globulinemia, chronic renal failure, alcoholism | →↑ | ↑↑ |
| V | Creamy top turbid bottom | Chylomicrons | Primary to familial mono-genic hypertriglyceridemia, apolipoprotein C-II deficiency<br>Secondary to uncontrolled diabetes, nephrotic syndrome, dysgamma- globulinemia, alcoholism | ↑ | ↑↑ |

Notes: IDL = intermediate-density lipoprotein; LDL = low-density lipoprotein; TC = total cholesterol; TG = triglycerides; VLDL = very-low-density lipoprotein ↑ = increased; ↑↑ = greatly increased; →= normal; →↑= normal or increased

*Source:* Adapted from Tietz NW. *Clinical Guide to Laboratory Tests*, 3rd ed. 1995.

**Table 13-4  Major Risk Factors That Modify Low-Density Lipoprotein Cholesterol***

Cigarette smoking
Hypertension (blood pressure ≥ 140/90 mm Hg or on antihypertensive medication)
Low level of high-density lipoprotein (HDL) cholesterol (< 40 mg/dL)[†]
Family history of premature coronary heart disease (CHD) (CHD in male first-degree relative < 55 years; CHD in female first-degree relative < 65 years)
Age (men ≥ 45 years; women ≥ 55 years)

* Diabetes is regarded as a coronary heart disease risk equivalent.
[†]HDL cholesterol ≥ 60 mg/dL counts as a "negative" risk factor; its presence removes one risk factor from the total count.

*Source:* National Cholesterol Education Program. Third Report of the Expert Panel on Detection, Evaluation, and Treatment of High Blood Cholesterol in Adults (Adult Treatment Panel III). ATP III At-A-Glance: Quick Desk Reference. Available at http://www.nhlbi.nih.gov/guidelines/cholesterol. Accessed January 20, 2010.

Table 13-5　**Low-Density Lipoprotein and Non-High–Density Lipoprotein Cholesterol Goals and Thresholds for Therapeutic Lifestyle Changes and Drug Therapy in Different Risk Categories**

| Risk Category | LDL Level at LDL Goal (mg/dL) | LDL Level at Which to Initiate Lifestyle Changes (mg/dL) | LDL Level at Which to Consider Drug Therapy (mg/dL) | Non-HDL Goal (mg/dL)* |
|---|---|---|---|---|
| CHD or CHD-risk equivalents: diabetes mellitus, atherosclerotic disease (CAD or stroke), or multiple risk factors (10-year risk > 20%) | < 100 | > 100 | ≥130 (100–129: drug optional)† | < 130 |
| 2+ risk factors: HDL < 40 mg/dL, strong family history, age > 45 years, and smoking (10-year risk > 20%) | < 130 | ≥ 130 | 10-year risk 10% to 20%: ≥ 130 10-year risk < 10%: ≥ 160 | < 160 |
| 0–1 risk factor‡ | < 160 | ≥ 160 | ≥ 190 (160 to 189: LDL-lowering drug optional) | < 190 |

Notes: LDL = low-density lipoprotein; CHD = coronary heart disease; CAD = coronary artery disease; HDL = high-density lipoprotein.

*Non-HDL cholesterol = (total cholesterol – HDL). When LDL cannot be measured because the triglyceride level > 200 mg/dL, non-HDL cholesterol may be used as a secondary goal. The non-HDL cholesterol goal is 30 mg/dL higher than the LDL cholesterol goal.

†Some authorities recommend use of LDL-lowering drugs in this category if an LDL cholesterol level < 100 mg/dL cannot be achieved by therapeutic lifestyle changes (dietary and exercise intervention). Others prefer use of drugs that primarily modify triglycerides and HDL (e.g., nicotine acid or fibrates). Clinical judgment also may suggest deferring drug therapy in this subcategory.

‡Almost all people with zero or one risk factor have a 10-year risk less than 10%; thus 10-year risk assessment in people with zero or one risk factor is not necessary.

Source: U.S. Department of Health and Human Services. National Guideline Clearinghouse. Prevention of Secondary Disease: Lipid Screening and Cardiovascular Risk. Available at www.guideline.gov/summary/summary.aspx?doc_id=10963. Accessed January 20, 2010.

Inhibition of HMG-CoA reductase lowers intracellular cholesterol levels, which causes an up-regulation of LDLRs. As a result, LDL-C clearance from the circulation is increased. As a group, the statins are generally well tolerated and have been well documented to lower cholesterol by as much as 25% to 50% below baseline. Statin doses required to attain an approximate 30% to 40% reduction in LDL-C levels have also been well established. Furthermore, the reduction of LDL-C in adults is directly proportional to a reduction of coronary events. For example, a sustained 5% reduction in LDL-C is equivalent to a 5% reduction in coronary events.

In some cases, statin treatment will cause an increase in liver enzymes (AST, ALT), so these enzyme levels need to be monitored for any abnormal elevation during treatment. Another adverse effect is muscle pain (especially in the lower legs); patients need to be educated to report such muscle pain, as there have been reported associations between statin use and rhabdomyolysis.

Cholesterol absorption inhibitors (e.g., ezetimibe) block intestinal absorption of cholesterol from the diet. This class of drugs has been shown to reduce LDL-C by 15% to 20% and is frequently used in conjunction with statins to reach target goals. Few side effects and relative safety yield a good compliance rate with these medications.

Bile acid–binding resins (e.g., colesevelam, colestipol) work by binding the cholesterol in bile acids in the intestines. Once bound, the cholesterol is not absorbed into the systemic circulation. The average cholesterol lowering effects achieved are between 10% and 20% of baseline. However, gastrointestinal side effects such as constipation, cramping, and bloating are common reasons for patient noncompliance.

Niacin produces a secondary reduction in LDL-C, but primarily functions to lower triglycerides (VLDL-C) and increase HDL-C. The LDL-C response occurs best at higher doses of the drug. Unfortunately, the adverse effects associated with niacin—such as pruritis, flushing, gout exacerbation, and peptic ulcer disease—contribute to decreased patient compliance. To reduce flushing, patients are advised to take a 325-mg aspirin 30 minutes before taking niacin and to take the medication with food (e.g., applesauce). Fibric acid derivatives also reduce synthesis of triglycerides (VLDL-C) and have been shown to reduce LDL-C between 10% and 15%, with some increase in HDL-C being noted as well. Although an increased risk of hepatitis and myositis has been reported in some patients who take these medications, the most common adverse reactions include elevated liver transaminases.

Recommended lifestyle changes for patients with dyslipidemia include smoking cessation, dietary changes (i.e., decrease consumption of fatty/fried foods, increase consumption of fruits and vegetables), weight loss, increased exercise, and management of diabetes mellitus and hypertension. The reduction of inflammation in the presence of chronic inflammatory diseases or infection is also beneficial. Dietary changes are a critical component of therapy for heterozygous FH, as they can reduce many risk factors and lower LDL-C levels. Increased consumption of dietary fiber is thought to help lower LDL-C by binding of the fiber with cholesterol in bile acids, thereby preventing the cholesterol from being absorbed in the gastrointestinal tract. Increased intake of monounsaturated fats such as olive oil may also reduce LDL-C oxidation. While increased physical activity primarily increases HDL-C and lowers serum triglycerides, it has also been shown to lower LDL-C levels. While many of these recommendations seem obvious for all patients—not just those with FH—in our current society it is very difficult for patients to adhere to them. Thus noncompliance is the greatest barrier to any of these suggested therapeutic lifestyle changes.

For healthcare providers, it is important to maintain a good working relationship with FH patients. This includes routine follow-up visits at least every 6 months. Given that most of the pharmacotherapeutic treatments for hyperlipidemia affect the liver, it is important to monitor not only fasting lipid profiles but also liver transaminases at least annually once desired blood cholesterol levels are achieved. Adjustments in medication doses may be necessary over the course of treatment, with each case being treated individually.

## Chapter Summary

- Familial hypercholesterolemia (FH) is characterized by increased levels of total serum cholesterol (hypercholesterolemia) with increased low-density lipoprotein cholesterol (LDL-C), tendinous xanthomata, and premature symptoms of coronary heart disease.

- Hypercholesterolemia is defined as a fasting total blood cholesterol level of more than 240 mg/dL.

- The LDL-C target goal is less than 100 mg/dL.

- Diagnostic tools for FH are not standardized, but often include a positive family history, clinical history of atherosclerotic disease, physical examination findings, blood cholesterol levels, and genetic testing for the LDLR gene.

- Several pharmocotherapeutic options are available to treat FH.

- Patients with FH should address modifiable risk factors such as poor dietary habits and smoking.

- Early diagnosis of FH can reduce the morbidity and mortality associated with this disease.

## Key Terms

**Allelic variant:** an alteration in the normal sequence of a gene.

**Angina:** chest pain that is precipitated by exertion and relieved by rest; it is caused by inadequate oxygen delivery to the heart muscles.

**Arcus corneus:** a corneal disease caused by deposits of phospholipids and cholesterol in the corneal stroma and anterior sclera surrounding the iris of the eye.

**Atherosclerosis:** thickening and loss of elasticity of arterial walls, caused by lipid deposition and thickening of the intimal cell layers within arteries.

**Cholesterol:** the principal sterol found in all higher animals. It is distributed in body tissues, especially the brain and spinal cord, and in animal fats and oils.

**Founder effect:** accumulation of random genetic changes in an isolated population as a result of its proliferation from only a few parent colonizers.

**Gain-of-function mutation:** a genetic change that increases the activity of a gene protein or increases the production of the protein.

**Loss-of-function mutation:** a genetic change that reduces the activity of a gene protein or decreases the production of the protein.

**Low-density lipoprotein:** the type of lipoprotein responsible for transport of cholesterol to extrahepatic tissues.

**Myocardial infarction:** death of the heart muscle, caused by occlusion of the coronary vessels.

**Xanthomas:** a cutaneous manifestation of lipid accumulation in the large foam cells that presents clinically as small eruptions with distinct morphologies along tendons such as the Achilles tendon.

**Xanthelasmata:** sharply demarcated yellowish collections of cholesterol in foam cells observed underneath the skin and especially on the eyelids.

## Chapter Review Questions

1. Familial hypercholesterolemia can result from a mutation in any of four genes: _____, _____, _____, or _____.

2. Familial hypercholesterolemia is characterized by increased levels of _____ and _____ and the physical examination findings of _____ and _____.

3. The target goal for LDL-C levels is _____.

4. The reduction of _____ in adults is directly proportional to the reduction of coronary events.

5. Thyroid abnormalities such as _____ are an important secondary cause of hypercholesterolemia.

## Resources

American Heart Association. www.americanheart.org.

Austin MA, Hutter CM, Zimmern RL, et al. Familial Hypercholesterolemia and Coronary Heart Disease: A HuGE Association Review. *American Journal of Epidemiology.* 160:421–429; 2004.

Austin MA, Hutter CM, Zimmern RL, et al. Genetic Causes of Monogenic Heterozygous Familial Hypercholesterolemia: A HuGE Prevalence Review. *American Journal of Epidemiology.* 160:407–420; 2004.

Daniels, SR, Greer, FR. Lipid Screening and Cardiovascular Health in Childhood. *Pediatrics.*122:198–208; 2008.

Gene Reviews. www.genetests.org.

Genetics Home Reference. http://ghr.nlm.nih.gov/.

Genetics Home Reference. Hypercholesterolemia. Available at: http://ghr.nlm.nih .gov/condition=hypercholesterolemia. Accessed January 27, 2010.

Goldstein JL, Hobbs HH, Brown MS. Familial Hypercholesterolemia. In Scriver CR, Beaudet AL, Sly WS, et al. (Eds.), *The Metabolic and Molecular Basis of Inherited Disease,* 8th ed. New York: McGraw-Hill; 2001, pp. 2863–2914.

Gotto A, Pownall, H. *Manual of Lipid Disorders,* 3rd ed. Philadelphia: Lippincott, Williams and Wilkins; 2003.

Grundy, SM, Cleeman, JI, Merz, NB, et al. Implications of Recent Clinical Trials for the National Cholesterol Education Program Adult Treatment Panel III Guidelines. *Circulation.* 110:227–239; 2004.

Leigh SE, Foster AH, Whittall RA, Hubbart BS, Humphries SE. Update and analysis of the University College London low density lipoprotein receptor familial hypercholesterolemia database. *Annals of Human Genetics.* 72:485–498; 2008.

Tietz NW. *Clinical Guide to Laboratory Tests,* 3rd ed. Philadelphia: W. B. Saunders; 1995.

# Chapter 14

# Hereditary Cardiomyopathies

## CHAPTER OBJECTIVES

✓ Describe the etiology and various forms of hereditary cardiomyopathies.
✓ Detail symptoms associated with hereditary cardiomyopathies.
✓ Discuss diagnostic criteria for hereditary cardiomyopathies.
✓ Discuss reduced penetrance.
✓ Review current surveillance and treatment recommendations for hereditary cardiomyopathies.

A **cardiomyopathy** is any condition in which the heart muscle (**myocardium**) is dysfunctional. Affected individuals are at increased risk for arrhythmias and sudden cardiac death. Cardiomyopathies are categorized based on the pathological features of the heart tissue itself. They may occur secondary to other diseases or may be hereditary in nature. This chapters discusses the two most common types of hereditary cardiomyopathies: familial hypertrophic cardiomyopathy (HCM) and arrhythmogenic right ventricular dysplasia or cardiomyopathy (ARVD/C).

Familial hypertrophic cardiomyopathy (formerly known as idiopathic hypertrophic subaortic stenosis) is characterized by unexplained **left ventricular hypertrophy** (LVH) that develops in the absence of other known causes. Mutations in various genes encoding for the contractile unit (**sarcomere**) of the heart muscle cells cause the muscle to be weakened, which impairs contractility. The clinical presentation of individuals affected by HCM may include dyspnea on exertion, palpitations, chest pain, and syncope. Some patients are asymptomatic, however. Unexplained LVH occurs in 1 in 500 persons. Known mutations in various sarcomere-associated genes are identifiable in approximately 70% of HCM cases.

Arrhythmogenic right ventricular dysplasia/cardiomyopathy is characterized by the replacement of normal heart muscle in the right ventricle by fibrous and fatty tissue. Similar to what happens with HCM, this abnormal tissue structure weakens the heart muscle and leads to impaired contractility. As in HCM, the clinical presentation of ARVD/C includes arrhythmias, palpitations, chest pain, and syncope. Incidence of ARVD/C has been reported to be 1 per 1000 persons in the overall population, with incidence reaching as high as 4.4 cases per 1000 population in the southern United States and in certain Mediterranean populations.

Both HCM and ARVD/C are associated with an increased risk for sudden cardiac death. Hypertrophic cardiomyopathy has been reported to be the leading cause of sudden cardiac death in competitive athletes in the United States, while ARVD/C is the second most common cause of sudden cardiac death and is more common in those younger than the age of 35. Both HCM and ARVD/C are inherited in autosomal dominant patterns.

## Diagnosis

Familial hypertrophic cardiomyopathy and ARVD/C can be difficult to diagnose. This challenge makes obtaining a thorough personal history and family history critical in patients being evaluated for fatigue, arrhythmias, palpitations, presyncope, syncope, or chest pain. Any of these physical symptoms in a person younger than the age of 35 or a positive family history of sudden cardiac death or unexplained death in first-degree relatives should raise the index of suspicion for HCM or ARVD/C. A family history of heart failure, hypertrophic cardiomyopathy, heart transplant, stroke, or blood clots is also important in this evaluation.

Physical examination findings in HCM may include extra heart sounds such as S4, prominent left ventricular apical pulse, apical lift, or brisk carotid upstroke. Abnormal electrocardiogram (ECG) findings are very common in both HCM and ARVD/C (**Figure 14-1**). The diagnosis of HCM is made based on a positive family history and/or molecular genetic testing in patients who have LVH in a nondilated ventricle as determined by echocardiography. The LVH must be present in the absence of predisposing factors such as hypertension or aortic stenosis. Although a myocardial biopsy can also establish the presence of LVH on the cellular level, this technique is usually reserved for autopsy.

The age of onset varies widely for HCM. Notably, LVH may become evident during the second decade of life (adolescence), with its development thought to be related to the onset of puberty. Development of LVH may occur as early as infancy and childhood, however, or it may not become apparent until later in life. This variation in the age of onset can occur within families and is thought to be due to variations in the phenotypic

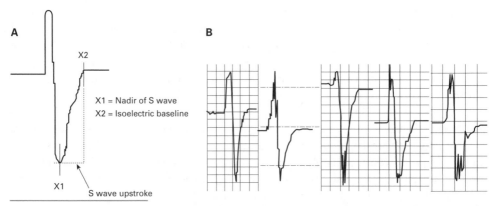

**Figure 14-1** Electrocardiogram findings associated with arrhythmogenic right ventricular dysplasia/cardiomyopathy. (A) Determination of an S-wave stroke from the QRS complex. (B) Examples of QRS complex in leads $V_1$ through $V_3$ from several ARVD/C cases demonstrating prolonged S-wave upstroke.

*Source:* Nasir K, Bomma C, Tandri H, Roguin A, et al. Electrocardiographic Features of Arrhythmogenic Right Ventricular Dysplasia/Cardiomyopathy According to Disease Severity: A Need to Broaden Diagnostic Criteria. *Circulation.* 110:1527–1534; 2004.

expression of the gene mutation. It also explains why some people who inherit the mutation do not develop the disease—a phenomenon known as reduced penetrance.

Four clinically observable phases of ARVD/C are distinguished. In the first, concealed phase, the person shows no clinical manifestations, but has a hidden risk of sudden cardiac death. This phase is followed by the development of symptomatic arrhythmias. In the third phase, right ventricular failure occurs. The fourth phase is marked by pump failure. It should be noted that left ventricular involvement can occur in any of the phases.

Although the physical examination is normal in at least 50% of patients with ARVD/C, one striking diagnostic clue is the presence of an extra heart sound such as a wide-split S2, S3, or S4. When the right ventricle is significantly dilated, asymmetry of the chest wall may be noticeable. Characteristic ECG findings are evident in as many as 90% of affected individuals (**Figure 14-2**) and have been incorporated into the major and minor diagnostic

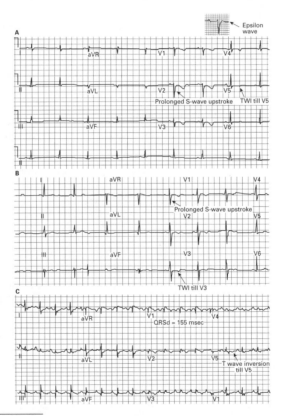

**Figure 14-2** Electrocardiograms from arrhythmogenic right ventricular dysplasia/cardiomyopathy (ARVD/C) patients. (A) Diffuse ARVD/C. (B) Localized ARVD/C. (C) ARVD/C with right bundle branch block pattern. (TWI = T-wave inversion).

*Source:* Nasir K, Bomma C, Tandri H, Roguin A, et al. Electrocardiographic Features of Arrhythmogenic Right Ventricular Dysplasia/Cardiomyopathy According to Disease Severity: A Need to Broaden Diagnostic Criteria. *Circulation.* 110:1527–1534; 2004.

criteria for ARVD/C (**Table 14-1**). Patients diagnosed with ARVD/C are typically between the ages of 19 and 45, and the majority are male.

Standard cardiac testing used in diagnosing cardiomyopathies such as HCM and ARVD/C includes a 12-lead ECG, signal-averaged ECG, exercise stress test, echocardiogram, cardiac MRI, and 24-hour Holter monitoring. Other tests, such as electrophysiological studies and myocardial biopsy, may be performed to complete the evaluation.

**Table 14-1  Major and Minor Diagnostic Criteria for Arrhythmogenic Right Ventricular Dysplasia/Cardiomyopathy**

Diagnosis requires either two major criteria, one major and two minor criteria, or four minor criteria from the following categories.

| Category | Major Criteria | Minor Criteria |
| --- | --- | --- |
| Global and/or regional dysfunction and structural alterations | Severe right ventricular dilation and reduction of right ventricular function with no (or only mild) left ventricular impairment | Mild global right ventricular dilation and/or ejection fraction reduction with normal left ventricle |
| | Localized right ventricular aneurysms (akinetic or dyskinetic areas with diastolic bulging) | Mild segmental dilation of right ventricle |
| | Severe segmental dilation of the right ventricle | Regional right ventricular hypokinesis |
| Tissue characterization of walls | Fibrofatty replacement of myocardium observed on endomyocardial biopsy | |
| Major repolarization abnormalities | | Inverted T waves in right precordial leads ($V_2$ and $V_3$) (age > 12 years, in absence of right bundle branch block) |
| Minor depolarization/ conduction abnormalities | Epsilon waves or localized prolongation (> 110 ms) of the QRS complex in right precordial leads ($V_1$–$V_3$) | Left bundle branch block-type ventricular tachycardia (sustained and nonsustained) on ECG, Holter monitor, or exercise testing |
| | Late potential (signal-averaged ECG) | Frequent ventricular extrasystoles (> 1000/24 h on Holter monitoring) |

*Continues*

Table 14-1   **Major and Minor Diagnostic Criteria for Arrhythmogenic Right Ventricular Dysplasia/Cardiomyopathy** (*Continued*)

| Category | Major Criteria | Minor Criteria |
|---|---|---|
| Family history | Familial disease confirmed at necropsy or surgery | Familial history of premature sudden death (< 35 years) suspected to be caused by right ventricular dysplasia |
| | | Familial history (clinical diagnosis based on present criteria) |

*Source:* Data from McKenna WJ, Thiene G, Nava A, Fontaliran F, et al. for the Task Force of the Working Group Myocardial and Pericardial Disease, the European Society of Cardiology and the Scientific Council on Cardiomyopathies of the International Society and Federation of Cardiology. Diagnosis of Arrhythmogenic Right Ventricular Dysplasia/Cardiomyopathy. *British Heart Journal.* 71:215–218; 1994.

## Genetic Testing and Counseling

As mentioned previously, ARVD/C and HCM are most commonly inherited in an autosomal dominant manner (McNally et al., 2009). New mutations in an individual (de novo mutations) are also transmissible to the offspring of that individual. Although its occurrence is rare, ARVD/C may also be inherited in an autosomal recessive pattern, especially in families from Greece. Some individuals have inherited multiple mutations. In these cases, evaluation should include an effort to determine the mode of inheritance through construction of a pedigree.

Eight genes are known to be associated with ARVD/C, whereas 12 different genes are linked to HCM. Testing of at-risk adult relatives for both disorders is routinely performed once the specific mutation has been identified in the proband. Unfortunately, mutation testing cannot predict the age of onset, constellation, or severity of symptoms. It can, however, identify those persons who require close surveillance. Screening guidelines have been proposed for asymptomatic relatives of the probands with HCM (**Table 14-2**). In particular, all first-degree family members of a proband with ARVD/C should undergo initial screening with the onset of puberty and have follow-up testing every 2 to 3 years.

## Management and Treatment

No treatment exists to prevent or delay disease expression for either HCM or ARVD/C. The primary goal of medical management is to prevent arrhythmias, syncopal episodes, and sudden cardiac death. Arrhythmias such as atrial fibrillation may initially be managed with pharmacologic therapies. Implantable cardioverter-defibrillators are indicated for

Table 14-2  **Screening Guidelines for Healthy Relatives of Probands with Familial Hypertrophic Cardiomyopathy**

| Age | Screening Guidelines |
|---|---|
| < 12 years | Optional but recommended, particularly if any of the following are present: family history of early HCM-related death, early development of LVH, or other adverse complications.<br>Competitive athlete in intense training program.<br>Symptoms: other clinical findings that suggest early LVH. |
| 12 to 18 years | Repeat evaluation every 12 to 18 months. |
| > 18 to 21 years | Repeat evaluation approximately every 3 to 5 years or in response to any change in symptoms.<br>Tailor the evaluation if the family has late-onset LVH or HCM-related complications. |

HCM = hypertrophic cardiomyopathy; LVH = left ventricular hypertrophy.
*Source:* Gene Reviews, www.ncbi.nlm.nih.

persons who have survived a cardiac arrest, are at high risk of cardiac arrest, or have arrhythmias that cannot be managed pharmacologically (e.g., sustained ventricular tachycardia). Persons who develop atrial fibrillation should receive anticoagulation therapy to prevent thromboembolism. Obstructive cardiac physiology in any person should be managed with prophylactic antibiotics to prevent endocarditis.

Pregnancy, even in stable patients, necessitates care by an obstetrician who specializes in high-risk pregnancies. Circumstances that patients should be advised to avoid include endurance training, burst activities, and isometric exercise. Patients with outflow obstruction should be encouraged to keep hydrated and cautioned about the use of diuretics, angiotensin-converting enzyme (ACE) inhibitors, angiotensin-receptor blockers, and medications used for erectile dysfunction.

Dyspnea in HCM is common due to diastolic dysfunction; beta blockers and calcium-channel blockers can be used to slow heart rate and improve this diastolic function by extending the filling period. Unfortunately, even with proper management, patients with cardiomyopathy often progress to heart failure. Heart transplantation remains a consideration when failure cannot be managed medically.

## Associated Syndromes

Left ventricular hypertrophy occurs in 1 in 500 persons, with almost 70% of all such cases being attributable to HCM. The remainder are due to either the associated syndromes discussed in this section or other, unknown causes.

Acquired left ventricular hypertrophy is found in competitive athletes who have undergone vigorous training. It may be distinguished from hereditary cardiomyopathies by observing whether a restriction imposed on physical training results in a decreased wall thickness of the myocardium.

Metabolic cardiomyopathy should be considered when LVH is found in conjunction with a pre-excitation syndrome such as **Wolff-Parkinson-White syndrome**.

As much as 10% of unexplained LVH in young adult males has been attributed to **Fabry disease**, an inherited lipid storage disease. Fabry disease results from a deficiency in the enzyme alpha-galactosidase found on the X chromosome. This defect leads to the accumulation of glycospingolipids in the plasma and lysosomes of vascular endothelial and smooth muscle cells. As a consequence, a fatty component of the cell wall cannot be broken down and builds up inside the cells, especially the cells lining the arteries and blood vessels. This accumulation of lipid clogs the blood vessels, which in turn damages the heart (heart attack) and kidneys (kidney failure). Lipid deposits are also found in cells of the cornea, kidney tubules, muscle fibers of the heart, and cells of the nervous system.

Cardiac amyloidosis is caused by deposition of an amyloid protein in the myocardium that displaces functional tissue. Normal cardiac movement is restricted by this buildup; thus this disorder is categorized as a "restrictive cardiomyopathy." Amyloidosis may be either inherited or occur as a de novo mutation.

Brugada syndrome is characterized by ST-segment abnormalities in leads $V_1$-$V_3$ on the ECG. This condition, which is associated with ventricular fibrillation and sudden cardiac death, most commonly occurs in young males of Asian descent.

Childhood cardiomyopathies have been associated with three major causes: inborn errors of metabolism, malformation syndromes, and neuromuscular disorders. The most common associated disorders in these categories are glycogen storage disease type II, Noonan syndrome, and Friedrich ataxia, respectively.

## Chapter Summary

- A cardiomyopathy is any condition in which the heart muscle (myocardium) is dysfunctional.

- Cardiomyopathies are categorized based on the pathological features of the heart tissue itself. They may either occur secondary to other diseases or be hereditary in nature.

- Familial hypertrophic cardiomyopathy is characterized by unexplained left ventricular hypertrophy that develops in the absence of other known causes.

- Arrhythmogenic right ventricular dysplasia/cardiomyopathy is characterized by the replacement of normal heart muscle in the right ventricle by fibrous and fatty tissue.

- Both familial hypertrophic cardiomyopathy and arrhythmogenic right ventricular dysplasia/cardiomyopathy are inherited in autosomal dominant patterns.

- No treatment exists to prevent or delay disease expression for these hereditary cardiomyopathies. Therefore, the primary goal of medical management is to prevent arrhythmias, syncopal episodes, and sudden cardiac death.

## Key Terms

**Cardiomyopathy:** any condition in which the heart muscle (myocardium) is dysfunctional.

**Fabry disease:** an inherited lipid storage disease that results from a deficiency in the enzyme alpha-galactosidase found on the X chromosome. This defect leads to the accumulation of glycospingolipids in the plasma and lysosomes of vascular endothelial and smooth muscle cells.

**Left ventricular hypertrophy (LVH):** enlargement of the muscle tissue in the wall of the left ventricle, often involving the intra-ventricular septum.

**Myocardium:** the heart muscle cells responsible for contractility of the heart.

**Sarcomere:** the simplest unit of muscle tissue that allows the muscle to contract.

**Wolff-Parkinson-White syndrome:** an electrocardiographic pattern sometimes associated with paroxysmal tachycardia; it consists of a short P-R interval (usually 0.1 second or less; occasionally normal) together with a prolonged QRS complex with a slurred initial component (delta wave).

## Chapter Review Questions

1. The majority of hereditary cardiomyopathies are attributed to _____ and _____.

2. The most life-threatening complications associated with cardiomyopathies are_____ and _____.

3. Both familial hypertrophic cardiomyopathy and arrhythmogenic right ventricular dysplasia/cardiomyopathy are inherited in an _____ pattern.

4. Signs and symptoms that raise clinical suspicion for familial hypertrophic cardiomyopathy include _____, _____, _____, and _____.

5. Electrocardiogram findings for arrhythmogenic right ventricular dysplasia/cardiomyopathy may include _____ and _____.

## Resources

Fabry Disease. http://www.fabrydisease.com/.

Hamid MS, Norman M, Quraishi A, Firoozi S, et al. Prospective Evaluation of Relatives for Familial Arrhythmogenic Right Ventricular Cardiomyopathy/Dysplasia Reveals a Need to Broaden Diagnostic Criteria. *Journal of American College of Cardiology.* 40:1445–1450; 2002.

McKenna WJ, Thiene G, Nava A, Fontaliran F, et al., for the Task Force of the Working Group on Myocardial and Pericardial Disease of the European Society of Cardiology and the Scientific Council on Cardiomyopathies of the International Society and Federation of Cardiology. Diagnosis of Arrhythmogenic Right Ventricular Dysplasia/Cardiomyopathy. *British Heart Journal.* 71:215–218; 1994.

McNally E, MacLeod H, Dellafave L. Arrhythmogenic Right Ventricular Dysplasia/Cardiomyopathy, Autosomal Dominant. *Gene Reviews.* 2009. Available at: http://www.ncbi.nlm.nih.gov/bookshelf/br.fcgi?book=gene&part=arvd. Accessed January 27, 2010.

Nasir K, Bomma C, Tandri H, Roguin A, et al. Electrocardiographic Features of Arrhythmogenic Right Ventricular Dysplasia/Cardiomyopathy According to Disease Severity: A Need to Broaden Diagnostic Criteria. *Circulation.* 110:1527–1534; 2004. http://circ.ahajournals.org/cgi/content/ full/110/ 12/ 1527.

Nava A, Bauce B, Basso, Muriago M, Rampazzo A, Villanova C, et al. Clinical Profile and Long-Term Follow-up of 37 Families with Arrhythmogenic Right Ventricular Cardiomyopathy. *Journal of American College of Cardiology.* 36:2226–2233; 2000.

Peters S, Trummel M, Koehler B, Westermann KU. The Value of Different Electrocardiographic Depolarization Criteria in the Diagnosis of Arrhythmogenic Right Ventricular Dysplasia/Cardiomyopathy. *Journal of Electrocardiology.* 40:34–37; 2007.

Sen-Chowdhry S, Syrris P, Ward D, Asimaki A, et al. Clinical and Genetic Characterization of Families with Arrhythmogenic Right Ventricular Dysplasia/Cardiomyopathy Provides Novel Insights into Patterns of Disease Expression. *Circulation.* 115:1710–1720; 2007.

*Stedman's Online Medical Dictionary.* http://www.stedmans.com/.

# Chapter 15

# Marfan Syndrome

## CHAPTER OBJECTIVES

✓ Describe the etiology and various forms of Marfan syndrome.
✓ Detail the phenotypic features, symptoms, and physical examination findings associated with Marfan syndrome.
✓ Discuss dominant negative mutation, variable expressivity, genetic heterogeneity, and genocopy.
✓ Review current treatment and surveillance recommendations for Marfan syndrome.

Marfan syndrome involves a defect of the connective tissue that is manifested as a series of disorders of multiple systems including the eye, aorta, and skin as well as overgrowth of the long bones. This syndrome results from either an inherited mutation or a new (de novo) mutation of the fibrillin-1 gene (*FBN1*). Phenotypically, these mutations are indistinguishable from each other. The heritable form follows an autosomal dominant pattern of inheritance, meaning that only one copy of the mutated gene is required to produce disease. De novo mutations produce disease in people without a positive family history of the disorder. While such cases are not as common as those involving inherited mutations, it is estimated that 25% of Marfan syndrome cases result from a new mutation in the *FBN1* gene. The incidence of Marfan syndrome ranges between 1 in 5000 and 1 in 10,000; it shows no obvious predilection by race, ethnicity, or gender.

## Phenotypic Features

Skeletal abnormalities often associated with Marfan syndrome include tall stature with long, thin arms and legs. Arachnodactyly (the presence of spider-like fingers) and an arm span exceeding the body height (dolichostenomelia) are also hallmark phenotypic features. An elongated, narrow face, a highly arched palate, overcrowded teeth, scoliosis, hyperflexible joints, and chest deformities are other common findings.

Ocular disorders associated with Marfan syndrome include myopia, the most common disorder, and lens displacement from the center of the pupil (ectopia lentis), which is observed in approximately 60% of affected individuals. Individuals with this disease are also at increased risk for retinal detachment, glaucoma, and early development of cataracts.

Abnormalities of the heart such as valve defects are often observed in people with Marfan syndrome and are the major cause of morbidity and mortality in affected individuals. The mitral valve and the aortic valve are the most commonly affected. Valvular insufficiency may manifest as palpitations, murmurs, shortness of breath, and fatigue. Weakening of the vessel wall of the aorta may result in stretching and lead to an aortic aneurysm or aortic dissection.

Stretching of the dural sac in the lumbosacral spine (dural ectasia), the development of bullae in the lungs, spontaneous pneumothorax, hernias, and stretch marks of the skin are other reported findings associated with Marfan syndrome. Pregnancy presents a special cause for concern and increased surveillance, as the risk for aortic dissection is increased in both the peripartum and postpartum stages.

Overall, there is a wide variation among affected individuals in regard to age at presentation, organ system manifestation, severity, and progression of the disease. Because physical findings tend to remain consistent among affected family members, however, the predominant determinate of phenotype is presumed to be the *FBN1* genotype.

## Genetics of Marfan Syndrome

The *FBN1* gene is the only known gene associated with Marfan syndrome. In normal individuals, this gene carries instructions for making the protein fibrillin-1, which has two main functions: (1) It combines with other structural proteins to form microfibrils, and (2) it regulates the growth and repair of various body tissues. **Microfibrils** are integral fibers that lend strength and flexibility to all connective, load-bearing tissues. Thus the characteristic features of Marfan syndrome created by the mutated *FBN1* gene are a product of dysfunction in each of these mechanisms. In addition, the mutated *FBN1* gene inhibits the production of the normal-functioning protein, blocking the formation of normal microfibrils (**dominant negative mutation**).

The specific *FBN1* mutations leading to Marfan syndrome vary widely among affected families and are often scattered across the gene (**genetic heterogeneity**). Because the penetrance of *FBN1* mutations is 100%, any offspring inheriting the mutated allele will develop Marfan syndrome, albeit with variable expressivity of the symptoms. **Variable expressivity** refers to the existence of variations in the symptoms associated with the disease. With Marfan syndrome, some affected individuals have multiple or severe symptoms, whereas others exhibit fewer or milder symptoms. It is important to note that the degree of severity in one affected individual will not dictate the degree of severity in that individual's offspring.

Marfan syndrome is inherited in an autosomal dominant pattern. Approximately 75% of affected individuals have an affected parent, while the remaining 25% cases involve random or de novo mutations. Therefore, the risk of inheriting the *FBN1* mutation and developing the syndrome is 50%.

## Diagnosis

Clinical diagnosis of Marfan syndrome is made based on both family history and the following physical examination findings: (1) aortic dilatation or dissection at the level of the sinuses of Valsalva, (2) ectopia lentis, (3) dural ectasia, and (4) four (of eight) specified skeletal features (**Table 15-1**). In patients for whom no family history is available, the criteria are adjusted to require major involvement in two systems and minor involvement in one other system.

Table 15-1 **Diagnostic Criteria for Marfan Syndrome**

| System | Major Criteria | Minor Criteria |
|---|---|---|
| Skeletal system | Presence of at least four of the following manifestations:<br>• Pectus carinatum<br>• Pectus excavatum requiring surgery<br>• Reduced upper-to-lower-segment ratio or arm span–to-height ratio greater than 1.05<br>• Wrist and thumb signs<br>• Scoliosis > 20 degrees or spondylolisthesis<br>• Reduced extensions at the elbows (< 170 degrees)<br>• Medial displacement of the medial malleolus causing pes planus<br>• Protrusio acetabulae of any degree (ascertained on radiographs) | • Pectus excavatum of moderate severity<br>• Joint hypermobility<br>• Highly arched palate with crowding of teeth<br>• Facial appearance (dolichocephaly, malar hypoplasia, enophthalmos, retrognathia, down-slating palpebral fissures) |
| Ocular system | • Ectopia lentis (dislocated lens) | • Abnormally flat cornea (as measured by keratometry)<br>• Increased axial length of globe (as measured by ultrasound) |
| Cardiovascular system | • Dilatation of the ascending aorta with or without aortic regurgitation and involving at least the sinuses of Valsalva<br>**or**<br>• Dissection of the ascending aorta | • Mitral valve prolapse with or without mitral valve regurgitation<br>• Dilatation of the main pulmonary artery, in the absence of valvular or peripheral pulmonic stenosis or any other obvious cause, before the age of 40<br>• Calcification of the mitral annulus before the age of 40 |

*Continues*

Table 15-1 **Diagnostic Criteria for Marfan Syndrome** *(Continued)*

| System | Major Criteria | Minor Criteria |
|---|---|---|
| | | • Dilatation or dissection of the descending thoracic or abdominal aorta before the age of 50 |
| Pulmonary system | None | • Spontaneous pneumothorax<br>• Apical blebs (ascertained by chest radiography) |
| Skin and integument | None | • Stretch marks not associated with marked weight changes, pregnancy, or repetitive stress<br>• Recurrent incisional hernias |
| Dura | • Lumbosacral dural ectasia diagnosed by CT or MRI | None |
| Family/genetic history | • Having a parent, child, or sibling who meets these diagnostic criteria independently<br>• Presence of a mutation in the *FBN1* gene known to cause the Marfan syndrome<br>• Presence of a haplotype around *FBN1*, inherited by descent, known to be associated with unequivocally diagnosed Marfan syndrome in the family | None |

*Source:* National Marfan Foundation. Diagnosis. Available at www.marfan.org/marfan/2319/Diagnosis#Criteria. Accessed January 20, 2010

## Genetic Testing and Counseling

Molecular genetic testing for *FBN1* mutations may be clinically useful to confirm a diagnosis, for prenatal diagnosis, and as predictive testing in families with known mutations. Clinical evaluation should include a medical history, thorough family history, and echocardiogram when there is high clinical suspicion for Marfan syndrome. Linkage analysis is available for those families in which a *FBN1* mutation has been previously identified.

## Management and Treatment

Today, the life expectancy of persons with Marfan syndrome approaches the life expectancy of the general population when cardiovascular risks are minimized. Cardiovascular surveillance should include annual echocardiograms. More frequent echocardiograms are recommended when the aortic root diameter is known to be enlarged above the threshold, when it exceeds the expected rate of enlargement on an annual basis, or when aortic regurgitation develops. Similar surveillance of the affected individual's relatives may also be indicated if clinical suspicion is raised by the person's phenotypic features or reported symptoms.

Affected individuals should be counseled to avoid contact sports, isometric exercise, caffeine, and decongestants due to increased stress that these factors place on the cardiovascular system. If individuals are found to be at increased risk for pneumothorax, they should be warned about the risks of breathing against resistance (such as playing brass instruments) and negative-pressure ventilation (e.g., scuba diving).

Annual eye examinations by an ophthalmologist are highly recommended to preserve vision. In addition to routine examination procedures, specific assessment for glaucoma and cataracts should be included in this monitoring. Any abnormalities should be managed by a specialist with experience in treating the ocular manifestations associated with Marfan syndrome. Severe scoliosis or other skeletal manifestations require the expertise of an orthopedist. Orthodontic evaluation is recommended particularly if the affected individual has a highly arched palate and/or overcrowded teeth.

Management and surveillance of Marfan syndrome are primarily aimed at early detection of symptoms and intervention to prevent disease progression. Recent studies suggest that losartan—an angiotensin receptor blocker used to treat hypertension—might eventually be used to prevent the clinical manifestations of Marfan syndrome. Losartan appears to inhibit aortic enlargement, reverses existing aortic root growth, and ameliorates lung and muscle tissue problems by blocking excess transforming growth factor-beta in mice models of Marfan syndrome.

## Associated Syndromes

Numerous other phenotypes are associated with mutations of *FBN1*, but do not meet the full diagnostic criteria for Marfan syndrome. Additionally, many of the characteristic skeletal features of Marfan syndrome are observed among the general population and may represent another underlying connective tissue disorder. Mitral valve prolapse syndrome may be present with variable expression of skeletal features. One specific phenotype associated with an *FBN1* mutation is known as MASS and involves myopia with mitral valve prolapse, aortic enlargement, and nonspecific skin and skeletal features. Aortic aneurysm, Marfanoid skeletal features, and familial ectopia lentis are all findings that the clinician must carefully differentiate from emerging Marfan syndrome.

Some genotypes, other than the *FBN1* mutation, can cause phenotypic features similar to those found in Marfan syndrome—referred to as **genocopy**. Examples include familial thoracic aortic aneurysms and aortic dissection (TAAD), Ehlers-Danlos syndrome, homocystinuria, and fragile X syndrome.

## Chapter Summary

- Marfan syndrome involves connective tissue defects that result in a multisystem disorder involving skeletal, cardiovascular, pulmonary, skin, ocular, and dural abnormalities.
- Marfan syndrome typically presents in early childhood.
- Marfan syndrome is a clinical diagnosis made based on family history and established findings across multiple organ systems.
- In this syndrome, mortality is related to cardiovascular disorders associated with this disease, such as aortic dissection.
- Surveillance guidelines include annual imaging of the aorta beginning in young adulthood.
- Pregnancy presents a special surveillance consideration, as women are at increased risk for aortic dissection and rupture.

## Key Terms

**Dominant negative mutation:** a mutated allele that disrupts the function of a normal allele in the same cell.
**Genetic heterogeneity:** the production of the same or similar phenotypes by different genetic mechanisms.
**Genocopy:** a genotype that determines a phenotype which closely resembles the phenotype determined by a different genotype.
**Microfibrils:** structural molecules found in load-bearing tissues.
**Variable expressivity:** variation in disease symptoms among persons with the same mutation.

## Chapter Review Questions

1. Marfan syndrome is the result of a mutation in the _____ gene.

2. _____ (the presence of spider-like fingers) and an arm span exceeding the _____ are hallmark phenotypic features of Marfan syndrome.

3. The most life-threatening complication associated with Marfan syndrome is _____.

4. The chance of an affected individual having offspring with Marfan syndrome is _____, which is described as _____ pattern of inheritance.

5. Physical examination findings that raise clinical suspicion for Marfan syndrome include abnormalities of the _____, _____, _____, _____, and _____ systems.

## Resources

De Paepe A, Devereaux RB, Dietz HC, et al. Revised Diagnostic Criteria for the Marfan Syndrome. *American Journal of Medical Genetics.* 62(4):417–426; 1996.

Dietz HC, Loeys B, Carta, LA, Ramirez F. Recent Progress Towards a Molecular Understanding of Marfan Syndrome. *American Journal of Medical Genetics Counselors Seminars in Medical Genetics.* 139(1):4–9; 2005.

Gene Reviews. www.genetests.org.

Genetics Home Reference. http://ghr.nlm.nih.gov/.

Gleb B. Marfan Syndrome and Related Disorders: More Tightly Connected Than We Thought. *New England Journal of Medicine.* 355(8):841–844; 2006.

Habashi JP, Judge DP, Holm TM, et al. Losartan, an AT1 Antagonist, Prevents Aortic Aneurysm in a Mouse Model of Marfan Syndrome. *Science.* 312:117–121; 2006.

Hiratzka LF, Bakris GL, Beckman JA, Bersin RM, Carr VF, Casey DE, et al. 2010 ACCF/AHA/AATS/ACR/ASA/SCA/SCAI/SIR/STS/SVM Guidelines for Diagnosis and Management of Patients 2ith Thoracic Aortic Disease: Executive Summary. *Circulation* 121;1544–1579; 2010.

National Marfan Foundation. www.marfan.org.

*Stedman's Online Medical Dictionary.* www.stedmans.com.

# Chapter 16

# Polycystic Kidney Disease

## CHAPTER OBJECTIVES

✓ Describe the etiology and forms of polycystic kidney disease.
✓ Detail symptoms associated with polycystic kidney disease.
✓ Discuss triplet repeat expansion and anticipation.
✓ Review current surveillance and treatment recommendations for polycystic kidney disease.

Polycystic kidney disease (PCKD) is a multisystem disorder that is most often characterized by bilateral renal cysts. While the most common cause of morbidity associated with PCKD is renal disease, intracranial aneurysms, aortic dissection and rupture, and cysts in other visceral organs are also known to occur. Polycystic kidney disease is caused by defects in the *PKD1* and *PKD2* genes, which encode for the membrane proteins polycystin-1 and polycystin-2, respectively.

Inheritance of PCKD most commonly follows an autosomal dominant pattern, in which it is known as autosomal dominant polycystic kidney disease (ADPKD). This variant is the most common potentially lethal single-gene disorder in the United States, with a prevalence of 1 case in every 500 people. It affects approximately 600,000 persons in the United States and 4 to 6 million people worldwide. Polycystic kidney disease may also follow an autosomal recessive pattern, in which case it is known as autosomal recessive polycystic kidney disease (ARPKD); this variant is relatively rare compared to ADPKD.

## Phenotypic Features

Polycystic kidney disease may be diagnosed in adulthood or childhood. depending on the severity of disease and its manifestations. Hypertension, flank pain, and renal insufficiency are the most common renal sequelae. All affected persons eventually develop cysts within the kidneys, but the number of cysts, the size of individual cysts, and the rate of progression are highly variable among individuals and within PCKD-affected families. The mutated gene product also varies, as noted in differences in signs between persons with mutations in *PKD1* versus *PKD2*. Specifically, at diagnosis, persons with *PKD1* mutations have larger kidneys with more cysts than those with *PKD2* mutations. This is due to earlier development of cysts in individuals with the *PKD1* mutation.

As multiple cysts and associated scarring replace the normal anatomic structures of the kidney, the usual renal physiological exchange processes—including filtration, reabsorption, and concentration of urine—are disrupted. In the presence of increased solutes and other favorable conditions, kidney stones may form. Renal perfusion may also become disturbed due to the structural changes in the cystic kidney. This problem usually precedes development of hypertension and may be clinically useful in early diagnosis given that most overt hypertension is detected late in the disease process. Long-standing hypertension can result in glomerular damage and kidney failure, aneurysms, cardiac valve disease, and complications during pregnancy for both the mother and fetus. Therefore, early detection allows for earlier treatment and ideally will prevent the emergence of cardiovascular disease, which is the main cause of death in these patients.

Flank pain, hematuria, proteinuria, kidney stones, and infections are common presenting features with this type of kidney disease. Factors that increase the risk of kidney stones in ADPKD are similar to the general risk factors for kidney stones—namely, decreased flow, increased solutes, and favorable pH for precipitation of solutes. The occurrence of these individual factors in ADPKD, coupled with structural changes within the kidneys stimulated by PCKD, contributes to increased prevalence of kidney stones in these patients. Most calculi in patients with ADPKD consist of uric acid with or without calcium oxalate, most likely due to decreased excretion of ammonia, acidic urinary pH, and decreased citrate concentration.

Females affected with ADPKD are more likely to develop urinary tract infections (UTIs) than their male counterparts. *Escherichia coli* and other enteric pathogens are the most common isolates of ascending infections. Such UTIs may progress to pyelonephritis and abscess-like infections of the renal cysts.

Progression to **end-stage renal disease** (ESRD) occurs in approximately 50% of adults with PCKD by the time they are 60 years of age. This outcome results from several different mechanisms, starting with the initial loss of functional renal tissue that has been replaced or compressed by the cysts. Over time, the vessels become sclerosed, inflammation occurs, and fibrotic tissue replaces functional tissue, causing further obstruction. Death of renal tubular epithelial cells is the final contributing feature in this process. Overuse of **nephrotoxic** medications, poor dietary habits, and concomitant chronic illnesses such as diabetes and hypertension are also detrimental to renal function.

Other complications associated with renal cysts include the development of aggressive cancer with ensuing compression of surrounding structures. While **renal cell carcinoma** occurs at the same frequency in patients with ADPKD as in the general population, it presents atypically and behaves more aggressively in ADPKD-affected individuals. As the kidneys become enlarged, nearby structures such as the intestines and inferior vena cava may become compromised.

Extra-renal manifestations may arise related to the liver, pancreas, seminal vesicles, arachnoid membrane, and spinal meninges. In fact, polycystic liver disease is the second most common finding associated with ADPKD. The incidence of liver (hepatic) cysts increases with patient age, with this sequala developing at a younger age among women with ADPKD than among affected males. Generally, these cysts are asymptomatic and do not parallel the problems observed with renal cysts. Rarely, the mass effect of liver cysts may cause abdominal distention with or without pain, fullness, decreased appetite, or pain on inspiration. The cysts may also compress nearby structures, such as vessels or bile ducts, leading to complications that may include bleeding, infection, or rupture.

Pancreatic cysts occur less frequently than renal or hepatic cysts in ADPKD patients and are usually discovered incidentally. They tend to be small and do not usually interfere with pancreatic function or cause complications.

Cysts of the seminal vesicles are mostly asymptomatic and occur in almost 40% of affected males without diminishing fertility. While arachnoid membrane cysts are usually asymptomatic, they may increase the risk of developing subdural hematomas.

The incidence of **diverticula** of the spinal meninges is slightly increased in persons with ADPKD, but the most life-threatening manifestation is the development of aneurysms. Intracranial aneurysms occur in 10% to 20% of persons affected with ADPKD, with the highest rates observed in individuals who have a positive family history of intracranial hemorrhage. Unlike in the general population, a history of renal dysfunction and hypertension does not usually precede the development of aneurysms in these families. In addition to diverticula of the meninges, **diverticulitis** of the descending colon is more prevalent in persons affected with ADPKD, especially after patients develop ESRD. Diverticular disease outside of the colon has also been reported.

Dilatation of the aortic root and cardiac valve abnormalities are associated with ADPKD as well. Aortic root dilatation may result in ascending aortic aneurysms that can propagate to involve the aortic arch and descending aorta. Recent evidence also suggests a link to thoracic aortic dissection. The most common valvular disorder is mitral valve prolapse, which is observed in 25% of affected individuals.

## Genetics

As mentioned earlier in this chapter, ADPKD is inherited in an autosomal dominant pattern. Thus persons with an affected parent have a 50% risk of inheriting the gene. Approximately 5% of all mutations involve de novo changes in the gene.

Polycystin-1 and polycystin-2 are proteins that are integral to specific membrane structures encoded by the *PKD1* and *PKD2* genes, respectively. When these genes are mutated, the protein complexes are rendered ineffective. These proteins are part of larger protein complexes located in the primary cilia of renal tubules, cardiac myocytes, and myofibroblasts of heart valves and vessels, which explains the multiple-organ system involvement that is characteristic of this disease.

Approximately 85% of disease expression is attributable to mutations of *PKD1*, with the remaining 15% due to *PKD2* mutations. Furthermore, mutations of *PKD1* tend to yield more severe clinical symptoms than mutations of *PKD2*. Persons with *PKD1* mutations are typically younger at presentation and have increased severity of renal disease with faster progression to ESRD. The expression of other organ system manifestations is the same with both mutations (**genetic heterogeneity**).

Environmental factors also influence disease expression. For example, hypertension before the age of 35, hematuria before the age of 30, hyperlipidemia at any age, and the coexistence of sickle cell trait all increase the likelihood and severity of PCKD.

Other factors that may contribute to disease expression include inherited genes that alter the expression of mutated genes (genetic modifiers). Some evidence also suggests that the position of the mutation leads to variability in disease expression. Homozygous expression is known to result in spontaneous abortion, usually in the second trimester of pregnancy.

Because the penetrance of disease is very high for PCKD, virtually all adults with mutations develop some level of disease. Notably, the penetrance of *PKD1* mutations is greater than that of *PKD2* mutations. Offspring of affected individuals are likely to have the same or greater level of disease as the affected parent. When the number of repeating units of the defective gene increases, the gene is expressed to a higher degree. This increase is called **triplet repeat expansion**, and the prediction of worsening expression of disease associated with it is termed **anticipation**.

## Diagnosis

Initial diagnosis of renal cysts is established by renal imaging, and the etiology of PCKD is later confirmed by genetic testing. Imaging studies are indicated in the scenario of asymptomatic presentation with a positive family history or when patients present symptomatically without a family history. Different diagnostic criteria for ADPKD exist for each group, as outlined in **Table 16-1**.

**Table 16-1   Diagnostic Criteria for Autosomal Dominant Polycystic Kidney Disease Based on Family History for Adults And Children**

| Type of Patient | No Family History* | Positive Family History |
|---|---|---|
| Adults | At least two unilateral or bilateral cysts in individuals younger than age 30 years | Enlarged kidneys noted on physical examination |
| | Two cysts in each kidney in individuals ages 30 to 59 years | Enlarged liver noted on physical examination |
| | Four cysts in each kidney in individuals age 60 years or older | Hypertension Mitral valve prolapse Abdominal wall hernia |
| Children | Large echogenic kidneys without distinct macroscopic cysts | |

*Sensitivity of 100% in individuals with autosomal dominant polycystic kidney disease who are older than 30 years of age and in younger individuals with *PKD1* mutations. Sensitivity is 67% for *PKD2* mutations in persons younger than 30 years of age.

*Source:* NCBI Bookshelf. Gene Reviews. Polycystic Kidney Disease, Autosomal Dominant. Available at www.ncbinlm.nih.gov.bookshelf/br.fcgi?book=gene&part=pkd-ad#pkd-ad.

When a parent is affected, his or her offspring should be clinically evaluated and undergo renal ultrasound to determine the presence and severity of cysts relative to patient age. In adult patients with ADPKD, the older the patient is at presentation, the more cysts he or she is likely to have compared to a younger patient (Table 16-1). The criteria given in Table 16-1 are 100% sensitive for patients with *PKD1* mutations who are older than the age of 30, but less sensitive for persons with *PKD2* mutations. In children, the PCKD-affected kidneys may appear enlarged and echogenic on ultrasound, but in most cases no cysts can be visualized.

When there is a positive family history of disease, a physical exam finding of enlarged kidneys or liver should raise the level of clinical suspicion for disease. Mitral valve prolapse, abdominal hernias, and hypertension in these patients are also indicative of disease. In persons without a family history of ADPKD, renal cysts—whether alone or in the presence of other findings (e.g., hepatic cysts)—is less considered less presumptive proof.

Imaging methods to identify and characterize cysts include abdominal ultrasound, computed tomography (CT), and magnetic resonance imaging (MRI). These techniques are also beneficial for examining extra-renal locations of disease, such as the liver. Even though imaging is an invaluable tool, diagnosis of PCKD is confirmed by molecular genetic testing.

## Genetic Testing and Counseling

Siblings of an affected proband have a 1 in 2 chance of being affected. Moreover, some affected individuals in the same family will become symptomatic before others. Testing for those at increased risk, including prenatal testing using amniotic fluid, is possible when the specific mutation has been identified in a family. Testing is also indicated for relatives of a proband in ESRD when screening relatives as candidates for a living-donor kidney transplant. Genetic counseling is indicated for those who are known to be affected or are considered at risk of PCKD due to a positive family history.

## Management, Treatment, and Surveillance

Initial treatment of PCKD depends on the disease manifestations at diagnosis. In addition to the usual lifestyle modifications to treat hypertension, renal-protective drugs such as angiotensin-converting enzyme (ACE) inhibitors or angiotensin II receptor blockers are prescribed. These drugs increase blood flow in the kidney—an effect that is particularly important for ADPKD-affected patients, who lose renal function when blood flow in the kidney is obstructed by cysts and associated scar tissue. ACE inhibitors and angiotensin II receptor blockers also have a relatively benign side-effect profile and have been shown to reduce development of arterial plaques (atherosclerosis), which might otherwise further complicate renal disease. A decrease in dietary protein consumption is also recommended for patients with PCKD to minimize glomerular damage and preserve renal function.

Routine evaluation after initial diagnosis of PCKD includes monitoring blood pressure, evaluating renal function and structure, evaluating liver structure, evaluating blood lipids, and screening for valvular and aortic disease (**Table 16-2**). Pain management may

**Table 16-2  Surveillance Recommendations for Persons Affected by Autosomal Dominant Polycystic Kidney Disease**

Renal ultrasound examination

Computed tomography (CT) imaging of the abdomen without and with contrast enhancement

Standardized blood pressure screening per recommendations of the American Heart Association

Measurement of blood lipids

Urine studies to detect the presence of microalbuminuria or proteinuria

Echocardiography or cardiac magnetic resonance imaging (MRI) to screen persons at high risk because of a family history of thoracic aortic dissections

Head MRI angiography or CT angiography to screen persons at high risk because of a family history of intracranial aneurysms

*Source:* NCBI Bookshelf. Gene Reviews. Polycystic Kidney Disease, Autosomal Dominant. Available at www.ncbinlm.nih.gov.bookshelf/br.fcgi?book=gene&part=pkd-ad#pkd-ad.

be needed for chronic flank pain associated with cysts and renal cystic changes. In severe cases, cysts may be removed or decompressed to alleviate the pain. Infected cysts require special attention and treatment with intravenous antibiotics. Screening for aneurysms is best accomplished by MRI.

A list of nephrotoxic drugs, including over-the-counter medications, should be provided to patients. Patients should be advised to avoid caffeine, as it may contribute to cyst growth. When there is liver involvement, patients should be warned about **hepatotoxic** agents as well. Because smoking damages the kidneys and independently increases the risk of renal cell carcinoma, efforts should be made to encourage smoking cessation as well as reduction of alcohol intake.

Recent clinical studies have focused on drugs that may help prevent cyst development and growth in PCKD. One drug being investigated for this purpose is octreotide, a synthetic form of somatostatin. While this drug's exact mechanism of action is not fully understood, it has been observed to reduce formation and growth of cysts.

## Associated Syndromes

Besides PCKD, there are no other known disorders associated with *PKD1* and *PKD2* mutations. However, numerous syndromes may present with renal cystic disease.

Autosomal recessive polycystic kidney disease is associated with bilateral renal cysts that have a different gross configuration as well as a distinct microscopic pathology from those observed in the autosomal dominant variant. Those persons affected with ARPKD do not have affected parents. Collectively, these features make ARPKD distinguishable from ADPKD.

Benign cystic kidney disease should be considered in the absence of a family history of ADPKD and when cystic disease is the only symptom. The prevalence of simple renal cysts increases with age, with such cysts being relatively rare in persons younger than age 50. Renal cysts are also associated with other disorders such as tuberous sclerosis complex, von Hippel-Lindau syndrome, oral–facial–digital syndrome type 1, glomerulocystic kidney disease, and Hajdu-Cheney syndrome. Differentiating these disorders from ADPKD depends on the constellation of symptoms and other organ systems that are involved.

## Chapter Summary

- Autosomal dominant polycystic kidney disease is a multisystem disorder that is most often characterized by bilateral renal cysts, intracranial aneurysms, aortic dissection and rupture, and cysts in other visceral organs.

- Autosomal dominant polycystic kidney disease is caused by defects in the *PKD1* and *PKD2* genes; it follows an autosomal dominant pattern of inheritance.

- Autosomal dominant polycystic kidney disease commonly manifests as hypertension, flank pain, and renal insufficiency in both children and adults.

- Diagnosis of autosomal dominant polycystic kidney disease requires renal imaging and may also include confirmatory genetic testing.

- While there is no cure for autosomal dominant polycystic kidney disease, treatment is targeted at preserving renal function by controlling hypertension and avoiding nephrotoxic agents.

## Key Terms

**Anticipation:** the predictability of progressively earlier onset and increased severity of certain diseases in successive generations of affected persons.

**Diverticula:** a pouch or sac opening from a tubular or saccular organ such as the intestines or the bladder.

**Diverticulitis:** inflammation of a diverticulum, especially of the small pockets in the wall of the colon, which fill with stagnant fecal material and become inflamed. Rarely, these sacs may cause obstruction, perforation, or bleeding.

**End-stage renal disease (ESRD):** the complete or almost complete failure of the kidneys to function. The dysfunctional kidneys can no longer remove wastes, concentrate urine, and regulate electrolytes.

**Genetic heterogeneity:** the character of a phenotype produced by mutation at more than one gene or by more than one genetic mechanism.

**Hepatotoxic:** relating to an agent that damages the liver.

**Nephrotoxic:** relating to an agent that damages renal cells.

**Renal cell carcinoma:** a type of kidney cancer in which the cancerous cells are found in the lining of very small tubes (tubules) in the kidney.

**Triplet repeat expansion:** a condition in which the number of repeating triplet units in a gene is so great that it interferes with gene expression and causes more severe disease.

## Chapter Review Questions

1. Autosomal dominant polycystic kidney disease is the result of a mutation in the _____ and _____ genes.

2. The main cause of morbidity in polycystic kidney disease is _____.

3. The most life-threatening complication associated with autosomal dominant polycystic kidney disease is _____.

4. The chance of an affected person having offspring with autosomal dominant polycystic kidney disease is _____, which describes an _____ pattern of inheritance.

5. Physical exam findings associated with autosomal dominant polycystic kidney disease include _____ and _____.

## Resources

Adeva M, El-Youssef M, Rossetti S, Kamath PS, Kubly V, Consugar MB, et al. Clinical and Molecular Characterization Defines a Broadened Spectrum of Autosomal Recessive Polycystic Kidney Disease (ARPKD). *Medicine (Baltimore)*. 85:1–21; 2006.

Belz MM, Fick-Brosnahan GM, Hughes RL, Rubinstein D, Chapman AB, Johnson AM, et al. Recurrence of Intracranial Aneurysms in Autosomal-Dominant Polycystic Kidney Disease. *Kidney International*. 63:1824–1830; 2003.

Ecder T, Schrier RW. Hypertension in Autosomal-Dominant Polycystic Kidney Disease: Early Occurrence and Unique Aspects. *Journal of the American Society of Nephrology*. 12:194–200; 2001.

Fain PR, McFann KK, Taylor MR, Tison M, Johnson AM, Reed B, Schrier RW. Modifier Genes Play a Significant Role in the Phenotypic Expression of *PKD1*. *Kidney International*. 67:1256–1267; 2005.

Gene Reviews. www.ncbi.nlm.nih. *Medline Plus Medical Encyclopedia*. http://www.nlm.nih .gov/medlineplus/ency/article/000500.htm.

National Kidney Foundation. www.kidney.org.

Qian Q, Harris PC, Torres VE. Treatment Prospects for Autosomal-Dominant Polycystic Kidney Disease. *Kidney International*. 59:2005–2022; 2001.

Rossetti S, Harris PC. Genotype–Phenotype Correlations in Autosomal Dominant and Autosomal Recessive Polycystic Kidney Disease. *Journal of the American Society of Nephrology*. 18:1374–1380; 2007.

*Stedman's Online Medical Dictionary*. http://www.stedmans.com/.

Torres VE, Harris PC. Mechanisms of disease: Autosomal Dominant and Recessive Polycystic Kidney Disease. *Nature Clinical Practice Nephrology*. 2:40–55; 2006.

Torres VE, Harris PC, Pirson Y. Autosomal Dominant Polycystic Kidney Disease. *Lancet.* 369:1287–1301; 2007.

U.S. Renal Data System. (USRDS). *USRDS 2002 Annual Data Report: Atlas of End-Stage Renal Disease in the United States.* Bethesda, MD: National Institutes of Health, National Institute of Diabetes and Digestive and Kidney Diseases; 2002.

Wang X, Wu Y, Ward CJ, Harris PC, Torres VE. Vasopressin Directly Regulates Cyst Growth in Polycystic Kidney Disease. *Journal of the American Society of Nephrology.* 19:102–108; 2008.

# Chapter 17

# Neurofibromatosis

## CHAPTER OBJECTIVES

✓ Describe the etiology and various forms of neurofibromatosis.
✓ Review the genetics associated with neurofibromatosis types 1 and 2.
✓ Provide diagnostic criteria for neurofibromatosis to
   assist the primary care provider.
✓ Detail current medical management options and
   recommendations for neurofibromatosis.

A **neurofibroma** is defined as a benign, encapsulated tumor resulting from proliferation of Schwann cells that are of ectodermal (neural crest) origin and that form a continuous envelope around each nerve fiber of peripheral nerves. The autosomal dominant genetic disorder known as neurofibromatosis (NF) causes such tumors to grow on the coverings of the nerves anywhere in the body at any time. This disorder affects 1 in 3000 to 4000 males and females of all races and ethnic groups worldwide and is one of the most common genetic disorders in the United States.

NF occurs in two distinctive forms: types 1 (NF-1) and 2 (NF-2). The most common form is type 1 NF, which manifests as tumors of the subcutaneous tissues and hyperpigmented skin lesions known as **café-au-lait spots**.

In NF, multiple neurofibromas may develop anywhere along the peripheral nerve fibers, from the roots distally. The resulting neurofibromas can become quite large, resulting in major disfigurement, bone erosion, and compression of various peripheral nerve structures. A small **hamartoma** (**Lisch nodule**) can be found in the iris of almost all patients. The effects of NF are unpredictable and have varying manifestations and degrees of severity (**Figure 17-1**).

NF type 2 has an incidence of 1 in 38,000 and occurs equally in males and females. This variant is characterized by the development of noncancerous tumors called **schwannomas** on the nerves that control hearing and balance (auditory and vestibular nerves). Although the tumors usually develop in late adolescence, some people do not develop problems until their forties and fifties. In the majority of cases, the schwannomas develop on both sides (bilateral) but not necessarily at the same time, so that there may be hearing loss of different degrees in the two ears. In some cases, schwannomas develop on only one side (unilateral) and other nerves may be affected by different types of tumors that control swallowing, speech, eye movements, and facial sensations. Tumors may also occur in the central nervous system (i.e., brain and spinal cord), but NF-2 has few cutaneous manifestations (**Figure 17-2**).

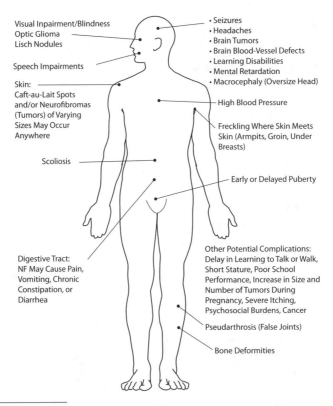

Visual Inpairment/Blindness
Optic Glioma
Lisch Nodules

Speech Impairments

Skin:
Caft-au-Lait Spots
and/or Neurofibromas
(Tumors) of Varying
Sizes May Occur
Anywhere

Scoliosis

Digestive Tract:
NF May Cause Pain,
Vomiting, Chronic
Constipation, or
Diarrhea

• Seizures
• Headaches
• Brain Tumors
• Brain Blood-Vessel Defects
• Learning Disabilities
• Mental Retardation
• Macrocephaly (Oversize Head)

High Blood Pressure

Freckling Where Skin Meets
Skin (Armpits, Groin, Under
Breasts)

Early or Delayed Puberty

Other Potential Complications:
Delay in Learning to Talk or Walk,
Short Stature, Poor School
Performance, Increase in Size and
Number of Tumors During
Pregnancy, Severe Itching,
Psychosocial Burdens, Cancer

Pseudarthrosis (False Joints)

Bone Deformities

**Figure 17-1** Body systems affected by neurofibromatosis type 1.
*Source:* Courtesy of Neurofibromatosis, Inc. Available at http://www.nfinc.org/nf1.shtml. Accessed August 13, 2010.

## Genetics of Neurofibromatosis

As mentioned previously, NF is an autosomal dominant genetic condition. Approximately 50% of those affected by this disease have a prior family history of NF; the other 50% appear to be the first members of their family to have the disorder. Two explanations for the latter situation are possible: (1) one of the parents actually does have NF-1, but its manifestations are so mild that he or she is unaware of it; or (2) neither parent has the disorder. However, if neither parent is affected, the mutation occurred in the sperm or egg. If individuals do not have NF, they cannot pass it on to their children.

Neurofibromatosis type 1, also called von Recklinghausen disease, is caused by a mutation in the *NF1* gene located on chromosome 17 that encodes for **neurofibromin**. The normal *NF1* gene is a **tumor suppressor gene** that probably suppresses activity of the ras protein following stimulation by nerve growth factor or other agents. Loss of tumor suppression due to *NF1* mutation presumably permits uncontrolled ras activation, which leads to the formation of neurofibromas.

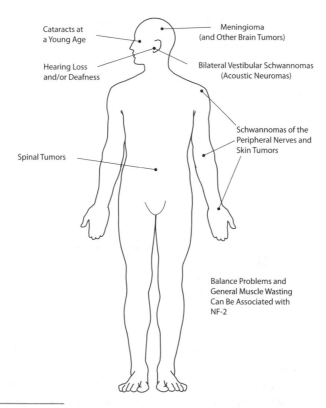

**Figure 17-2** Body systems affected by neurofibromatosis type 2.
*Source:* Courtesy of Neurofibromatosis, Inc. Available at http://www.nfinc.org/nf2.shtml. Accessed August 13, 2010.

While there appear to be similarities between NF-1 and NF-2, evidence of distinct origins exists for each. Type 2 NF is also characterized by autosomal dominant inheritance, and is caused by mutation in the *NF2* gene on chromosome 22 that encodes for **merlin**. Because merlin is also a tumor suppressor gene, the NF-related mutation disrupts this activity and leads to the formation of schwannomas.

Even though the genes for both NF-1 and NF-2 have been identified, there is no known cure for either form of NF.

## Diagnosis

While mutation analysis is 60% to 70% accurate in detecting the mutations associated with NF-1 and NF-2, this type of genetic testing is not widely available. As a consequence, a family history (even though 50% of patients diagnosed with NF are the first in their family to have this disorder) and a thorough physical examination are needed to diagnose NF. Generally, most individuals who develop NF are not born with café-au-lait macules; rather,

## Table 17-1  Diagnostic Criteria for Neurofibromatosis Type 1

Two or more of the following must be present:

1. 1.5 cm or larger in postpubertal individuals; six or more café-au-lait spots 0.5 cm or larger in prepubertal individuals

2. Two or more neurofibromas of any type or one or more plexiform neurofibroma

3. Freckling in the axillary or inguinal region

4. Optic glioma (tumor of the optic pathway)

5. Two or more Lisch nodules (benign iris hamartomas)

6. A distinctive bony lesion: dysplasia of the sphenoid bone or dysplasia or thinning of long bone cortex

7. A first-degree relative with neurofibromatosis type 1

*Source:* Adapted from Neurofibramatosis. *NIH Consensus Statement Online.* 1987. July 13–15 [cited November 14, 2009]; 6(12): 1–19. http://consensus.nih.gov/1987/1987Neurofibromasis064 html.htm and http://www.nfinc.org/nf1.shtml.

these skin lesions develop during the first 3 years of life and prompt parents to seek medical attention for their child. Neurofibromas start to form in late adolescence. **Table 17-1** lists the diagnostic criteria for NF-1.

The presence of multiple café-au-lait spots strongly suggests—but does not prove—the diagnosis of NF-1. In rare cases, individuals may have as many as six café-au-lait spots, yet not exhibit other features of NF-1. In children between the ages of 5 and 12, the presence of café-au-lait macules greater than 0.5 cm in diameter is highly suggestive of NF; it is recommended that further testing be pursued in these children. While healthy individuals may have one or two macules of this kind, children with three or more macules should be worked up. Because many features associated with NF-1 may not appear until late childhood or adolescence, it is often impossible to make a definitive diagnosis of NF-1 in a young child whose only manifestations are multiple café-au-lait spots. Even if the child is affected, it could take years before another feature of the disorder appears and confirms the diagnosis. Consequently, healthcare providers should reexamine these children to look for the appearance of new features on an annual basis. If any are found, the diagnosis is clear; if not, the question remains unsettled.

Lisch nodules are dome-shaped hamartomas of the iris that are found superficially around the eyes on slit lamp examination. Although asymptomatic, their presence helps in confirming the diagnosis of NF. Axillary freckling (as well as freckling on the perineum), known as the **Crowe sign**, is another helpful diagnostic feature in NF. Both axillary freckling and inguinal freckling often develop during puberty. Areas of freckling and regions of **hypertrichosis** occasionally overlay plexiform neurofibromas, which are often large,

Table 17-2   **Diagnostic Criteria for Neurofibromatosis Type 2**

**Confirmed (Definite) Neurofibromatosis Type 2**

1. Bilateral vestibular schwannomas (VS; also known as acoustic neuroma)

**Presumptive (Probable) Neurofibromatosis Type 2**

1.  Family history of neurofibromatosis type 2 (first-degree family relative) plus:

2.  Unilateral VS or any two of the following:
    • Meningioma
    • Posterior subcapsular lenticular opacity
    • Glioma
    • Cortical cataract
    • Schwannoma

**Individuals with the following clinical features should be evaluated for neurofibromatosis type 2:**

1.  Unilateral VS plus at least two of any of the following: meningioma, glioma, schwannoma, juvenile posterior subcapsular lenticular opacities/juvenile cortical cataract

2.  Multiple meningiomas (two or more) plus unilateral VS or any two of the following: glioma, schwannoma, juvenile posterior subcapsular lenticular opacities/juvenile cortical cataract

*Source:* Adapted from Neurofibramatosis. *NIH Consensus Statement Online.* 1987. July 13–15 [cited November 14, 2009]; 6(12): 1–19. http://consensus.nih.gov/1987/1987Neurofibromasis064 html.htm and http://www.nfinc.org/nf2.shtml.

infiltrative tumors that cause severe disfigurement of the face or an extremity. Bone involvement can include pseudoarthrosis of the tibia, bowing of the long bones, and orbital defects. Mild scoliosis may be encountered, and localized hypertrophy of bone, especially on the face, may be identified. Whether these bone changes are caused by diffuse neurofibromas or other kinds of mesodermal defects is not entirely clear. **Gliomas** of the optic nerve may also occur.

Neurofibromas are classified into one of three categories according to their gross pathology: (1) cutaneous, (2) subcutaneous, or (3) plexiform. They vary from brown to pink or flesh in color and may be either soft or firm to palpation. Various central nervous system tumors (e.g., astrocytomas, meningiomas, intramedullary gliomas, and ependymomas) occur with greater frequency in these patients. Any of these tumors may manifest as seizures, increased intracranial pressure, ataxia, or cranial nerve pathologies. In NF-2, schwannomas are the most common tumor and involve cranial and peripheral nerves (**Table 17-2**).

The incidence of learning disabilities and mental retardation among persons with NF-1 is as high as 40% and 10%, respectively. Common learning disabilities include neuromotor dysfunction, attention–deficit/hyperactivity disorder, and visuospatial processing disorders. In addition, endocrine disorders, short stature, and growth hormone deficiency are noted to coexist in a higher-than-normal prevalence in this population.

## Medical Management

Because there is no cure for NF-1 or any medical or surgical treatment that can reverse or prevent most related complications, medical management of NF-1 is limited to early detection of treatable complications. Examples of such care include assessment and management of learning disabilities or surgery referral to remove or reduce the size of neurofibromas. Anticipation of such problems and prompt intervention can greatly improve the outcome of treatment.

A person with NF-1 should have a complete medical evaluation at least once a year, to be conducted by a healthcare provider who is familiar with this disorder. During this evaluation, the provider should update the medical history as well as perform physical, neurological, and ophthalmologic examinations. Careful attention should be paid to any new signs or symptoms of NF-1, especially changes in skin manifestations such as growth of or pain in a neurofibroma. If specific problems are found, referral should be made to appropriate medical consultants or specialists for assistance. In the pediatric patient, cognitive development and school progress should be discussed, as early identification of potential learning disabilities related to NF-1 is essential for proper intervention.

In general, any signs or symptoms of neurological problems should be fully investigated, including ordering a CT or MRI scan of the brain. In patients suspected of having NF-2, MRI of the head is recommended in early adolescence. The value of such a scan in the absence of signs or symptoms of neurological impairment is not as clear, however, and different medical providers may make different recommendations. Some providers see these additional tests as a way to obtain as complete a picture as possible of a person's NF-1, whereas others believe that they are unnecessary in the absence of symptoms given the likelihood that nothing treatable would be found. It has been suggested that healthcare providers have an open discussion with patients and their families regarding the risks, benefits, and costs associated with these screening tests.

Regular slit lamp eye examinations are also an important part of managing NF-1. The presence of Lisch nodules can help in establishing a diagnosis of NF-1, so the primary care provider should consider referral to an ophthalmologist in suspected patients. Lisch nodules are not medically significant and do not interfere with vision, but complications relating to optic glioma, or problems with bone structure behind the eye, such as the orbit, may occur in people with NF-1. Other recommendations for specialist referral are shown in **Table 17-3**.

**Table 17-3 Recommendations for Specialist Referral For Neurofibromatosis Patients**

| Disorder | Specialist |
| --- | --- |
| Tibial bowing | Orthopedic surgeon |
| Skin (especially facial) deformities | Plastic surgeon |
| Self-esteem issues, language disorders, learning disabilities | Psychiatrist/psychologist |
| Hearing deficit | Ears, nose, and throat specialist |

# Chapter Summary

- The autosomal dominant genetic disorder known as neurofibromatosis causes tumors to grow on the covering of the nerves anywhere in the body at any time.

- Type 1 neurofibromatosis is the most common variant of this disease; it is characterized clinically by the combination of patches of hyperpigmentation and cutaneous and subcutaneous tumors.

- Type 2 neurofibromatosis is characterized by the development of noncancerous tumors called schwannomas on the nerves that control hearing and balance.

- Neurofibromatosis type 1, also called von Recklinghausen disease, is caused by a mutation in the *NF1* gene located on chromosome 17, which encodes for neurofibromin.

- Type 2 neurofibromatosis is caused by a mutation in the *NF2* gene located on chromosome 22, which encodes for merlin.

- There is no cure for type 1 neurofibromatosis, so medical management is limited to the early detection of treatable complications.

# Key Terms

**Café-au-lait spot:** a flat spot on the skin that is the color of coffee with milk (café au lait) in persons with light skin. These spots are harmless by themselves, but in some cases they may be a sign of neurofibromatosis. The presence of six or more café-au-lait spots, each of which is 1.5 centimeters or more in diameter, is diagnostic for neurofibromatosis.

**Crowe sign:** axillary and inguinal freckling, often associated with type 1 neurofibromatosis.

**Glioma:** any neoplasm derived from one of the various types of cells that form the interstitial tissue of the brain, spinal cord, pineal gland, posterior pituitary gland, and retina.

**Hamartoma:** a focal malformation that resembles a neoplasm, grossly and even microscopically, but results from faulty development in an organ.

**Hypertrichosis:** growth of hair in excess of the normal.

**Lisch nodule:** iris hamartomas, typically seen in type 1 neurofibromatosis.

**Merlin:** a tumor suppressor gene encoded on chromosome 22 (*NF2* gene). Mutation of this gene disrupts tumor suppressor activity and leads to the formation of schwannomas associated with type 2 neurofibromatosis.

**Neurofibroma:** a benign, encapsulated tumor resulting from proliferation of Schwann cells that are of ectodermal (neural crest) origin and that form a continuous envelope around each nerve fiber of peripheral nerves.

**Neurofibromin:** a tumor suppressor gene encoded on chromosome 17 (*NF1* gene). Loss of tumor suppression due to a mutation in this gene leads to the formation of neurofibromas associated with type 1 neurofibromatosis.

**Schwannoma:** a benign, encapsulated neoplasm in which the fundamental component is structurally identical to a syncytium of Schwann cells. The neoplasm may originate from a peripheral or sympathetic nerve, or from various cranial nerves, particularly the eighth nerve.

**Tumor suppressor gene:** a gene that encodes a protein involved in controlling cellular growth; inactivation of this type of gene leads to deregulated cellular proliferation, as in cancer.

## Chapter Review Questions

1. _____ neurofibromatosis is the most common and is characterized clinically by the combination of patches of hyperpigmentation and cutaneous and subcutaneous tumors.

2. Type 2 neurofibromatosis is characterized by the development of noncancerous tumors called _____ on the nerves that control hearing and balance.

3. Loss of tumor suppression due to *NF1* mutation presumably permits uncontrolled _____, which leads to the formation of neurofibromas.

4. The presence of multiple café-au-lait spots proves a patient has type 1 neurofibromatosis: True or false?

5. Neurofibromatosis is an _____ genetic condition, and approximately 50% of those affected have a prior family history of this disorder.

## Resources

Dermatology Image Atlas. http://dermatlas.med.jhmi.edu/derm/index.cfm.

Kam JR, Helm TH. Neurofibromatosis. 2008. http://emedicine.medscape.com/ article/ 1112001-overview.

MedicineNet.com. http://www.medterms.com/script/main/hp.asp.

Neurofibromatosis. *NIH Consensus Statement Online.* 6(12):1–19; July 13–15, 1987 [cited November 14, 2009].

Neurofibromatosis, Inc. http://www.nfinc.org/.

Neurofibromatosis Type 2. Centre for Genetics Education, *Fact Sheet 52.* Updated June 2007. http://www.genetics.com.au/factsheet/fs52.html

*Stedman's Online Medical Dictionary.* http://www.stedmans.com/.

Understanding NF1. http://www.understandingnf1.org/id/int_id_win.html.

# Chapter 18

# Familial Malignant Melanoma

## CHAPTER OBJECTIVES

✔ Describe the etiology and various forms of familial malignant melanoma.
✔ Detail symptoms associated with familial malignant melanoma.
✔ Discuss gene penetrance, variable expressivity, and skin phototype.
✔ Review the current surveillance, diagnosis, and treatment recommendations for familial malignant melanoma.

Malignant melanoma (MM) originates from melanocytes, the pigment-producing cells commonly found in the basal layer of the skin's epidermis. This type of cancer affects approximately 59,940 persons per year in the United States, causing 8110 deaths per year, and represents the sixth-leading cause of cancer incidence in this country. The lifetime probability of developing MM is 1 in 49 for men and 1 in 73 for women. Over the last 30 years, incidence of MM has been on the rise in young men (younger than age 30 years), with an increasing death rate from this cause being observed among this age group. This disease occurs sporadically in 80% to 90% of cases, with familial patterns being observed in the remaining 10% to 20% of cases. Because MM exhibits early metastasis and shows poor response to treatment once it has progressed, its emergence qualifies as a health crisis. Both environmental and genetic factors are involved in the development of melanoma (**melanomagenesis**).

Melanoma occurring in the familial pattern known as familial atypical multiple mole and melanoma (FAMMM) syndrome, also known as dysplastic nevus syndrome (DNS) and atypical mole syndrome (AMS), is characterized by the appearance of a large number of dysplastic nevi or atypical moles at an early age in combination with MM. The term "atypical" describes the gross appearance of the mole on visual examination, while "dysplastic" refers to the microscopic appearance of the tissue from biopsy. When MM does occur in these patients, they exhibit a more aggressive disease progression than is observed with sporadic melanoma, most likely due to higher gene **penetrance**.

## Environmental Factors

Although the reason for the increased incidence of MM is unclear, exposure to ultraviolet (UV) radiation is almost certainly a contributing factor. In particular, sunburns and childhood exposure to UV rays are known to increase a person's risk of developing MM. In addition, certain aspects of UV light may affect overall survival from MM. Intensity of UV light is also a factor in development of MM, as evidenced by the geographical patterns

**Table 18-1   Phenotypic Features Predictive of Risk for Malignant Melanoma**

Light complexion and inability to tan

Red hair

Number of atypical nevi greater than or equal to 10

Anatomic location of atypical nevi (especially back)

Freckles

---

of MM that occur relative to equatorial latitude. Ultraviolet radiation is thought to play a role in melanomagenesis among MM families by affecting gene penetrance. Furthermore, UV exposure may play an additive role in MM families, as it tends to be a common environmental factor among kindreds.

## Phenotypic Features

Physical characteristics have been reported in numerous studies to infer a higher risk of MM, regardless of genotype or family history (**Table 18-1**). These associated risk factors include light skin color, **phototype** (ability to tan), hair color, number of freckles, number of atypical nevi, and anatomical distribution pattern of atypical nevi. Red hair and freckles are associated with the *MC1R* gene, which has also been shown to predispose individuals to MM. This gene association with MM is present even in the absence of red hair, making both freckles and red hair independent phenotypic risk factors for MM. Atypical nevi are well-documented precursors to MM. Studies have suggested that AMS and DNS are associated with FAMMM syndrome and are seen in approximately 15% of the general population. Multiple moles and positive family history are also well-known risk factors for developing MM, as dysplastic nevi occur as precursors in familial patterns of MM. These "atypical moles" have been found to be related to an autosomal dominant trait encoded on chromosome 9p16.

An increased number of atypical nevi and the anatomical distribution of nevi are independent risk factors for MM. A finding of more than 100 nevi or six or more dysplastic nevi is significantly associated with a family history of melanoma. In addition, some melanoma-affected families show aggregation of phenotypes for factors such as number of nevi and skin phototype. These phenotypes may be associated with MM independent of shared genes and common environmental exposures among family members.

## Genetics

In studies of families where multiple cases of melanoma have developed among kindreds, the chromosomal region 9p21 has been implicated as a causative factor. In addition to this locus, some other gene sets appear to be involved in the process of nevi differentiation into melanoma. Various mutations in four specific genes (*CDKN2A, CDK4, p14ARF,* and *MC1R*) have been identified in only some of these known familial cases, however; the etiologies of the remaining cases are currently unknown. Even though **variable expressivity** and gene penetrance are thought to play a partial role in disease expression among mutation carriers, interaction between **covariates** and melanoma genes is also suspected.

The FAMMM or AMS phenotypes have been associated with specific genetic mutations, but it is important to note that these phenotypes alone are not indicators of mutation status. Because the absence of these genetic mutations does not confer a decreased risk in MM families, it is probable that familial MM involves the interplay of environmental factors with genetic predisposition. Phenotypic expression has also been shown to vary among MM-affected families depending on ancestry (i.e., British, Swedish, Italian, Brazilian, or Scottish families).

## Diagnosis

When accurately reported, family history is the most reliable indicator of risk for MM, regardless of mutation status (**Table 18-2**). Barriers to obtaining an accurate family history may include an unknown biological family history, inability of patients to differentiate between melanoma and non-melanoma skin cancers, and a fear of having an unfavorable medical history appear in the medical record. Not only have patients with more than two family members with MM been found to be more likely to develop MM themselves, but the disease also has an earlier age of onset in these individuals and tends to produce multiple primary lesions. While all first- and second-degree relative occurrences of MM are considered significant risk factors, the greatest familial risk indicator is a parent affected by multiple primary melanomas. The need to collect a detailed extensive family history at the initial visit followed by annual review and updates cannot be overstated.

Melanoma can occur anywhere on the body. In males, it is more frequently found on the trunk, head, and neck, whereas females tend to develop melanoma predominantly on the arms and legs. Changes in the appearance of a mole or pigmented lesion may be a sign of melanoma. If a mole or pigmented area of skin changes or looks abnormal, complete

---

**Table 18-2   Pertinent Family History Predictive of Risk for Malignant Melanoma**

Malignant melanoma in first- or second-degree relatives

Malignant melanoma of more than three occurrences among any family members

Malignant melanoma with multiple primaries in one parent

Malignant melanoma with multiple primaries in any one individual

Malignant melanoma with multiple cases on same side of family

Malignant melanoma diagnosed in family member at young age

Pancreatic adenocarcinoma

Breast cancer

Central nervous system cancers

Non-melanoma skin cancer

skin examination by a qualified healthcare provider should be performed (National Cancer Institute, Melanoma Treatment [PDQ®], 2010). Suspicious lesions can be biopsied to remove as much of the lesion as possible. The tissue is then examined microscopically by a pathologist to detect cancer cells. Such lesions should never be shaved, frozen, cauterized, or removed with a laser.

Any mole that exhibits changes in size, shape, or color; has irregular borders; or demonstrates asymmetry should be evaluated by a dermatologist. Lesions that itch, have discharge, or bleed are also cause for concern. Any lesion that forms **satellite moles** or moles that grow in a pattern around existing moles are also highly suspicious.

Staging takes into consideration both the characteristics of the original melanoma and metastasis (i.e., the degree to which the primary cancer has spread to lymph nodes or other organs). Staging is required to develop the appropriate treatment plan. Approaches used in staging include **wide local excision**, **lymph node mapping**, various imaging studies, and laboratory assays. Wide local excision involves removal of some normal tissue surrounding the area of the primary melanoma. This tissue is then examined microscopically to determine whether melanoma cells are present. If any cancer cells remain, the excision is widened to ensure that no melanoma remains at the primary site.

Clark's levels are used to classify thin tumors in terms of how deep the cancer has spread into the skin. Tumors may be confined to the epidermis (Clark's level I), spread into different depths of the dermis (Clark's levels II, III, and IV), or spread into subcutaneous tissue (Clark's level V).

Lymph node mapping with sentinel lymph node biopsy is a procedure in which a radioactive substance or a dye is injected near the tumor (National Cancer Institute, Breast Cancer Treatment [PDQ®], 2010). The substance flows through the lymph system and into the first major lymph node (**sentinel node**), which is the most likely location where cancer cells have spread. The nodes that are "mapped" are then removed and examined microscopically for evidence of cancer cells. If no cells are detected in the sentinel node, it is not necessary to remove the remaining lymph nodes in this area. Other diagnostic tests include a chest x-ray to screen for lung and bone metastases. **Computed tomography (CT) scans** of the chest, abdomen, and pelvis are also usually performed, while **magnetic resonance imaging (MRI)** is the preferred scanning modality for gross observation of brain metastases. The detection of smaller metastases requires a full-body **positron emission tomography (PET) scan**. This imaging procedure detects glucose uptake by cancer cells—such cells have a faster metabolic rate than noncancerous cells. It should be noted that PET scans are able to detect smaller tumors (micrometastases) that are not identifiable through other imaging studies.

The laboratory assay most commonly used in staging is serum lactate dehydrogenase (LDH). This enzyme is found in the cells of many tissues, such as the lungs, liver, kidneys, skeletal muscles, and brain. When injury (such as invasion by a tumor) occurs in these tissues, LDH is released in greater quantity into the serum. Because this enzyme is found in many tissues, however, an increase in total LDH is not very specific. Nevertheless, LDH is relatively sensitive for solid-tumor malignancies and its level may be significantly elevated when cancer cells are present. These characteristics make LDH a good screening tool for detecting occult metastases.

More recently introduced staging systems take into account other factors that are independent variables for prognosis. The overall thickness of the primary tumor (both above and below the epidermis) is considered more important than the Clark's level, for example. The presence of ulceration in the primary tumor and the number of lymph nodes involved are also more valuable information than the size of positive lymph nodes. Elevated serum LDH in stage IV disease is a negative prognostic indicator.

## Genetic Testing and Counseling

In general, dermatologists and other clinicians agree that testing should not be routinely performed for specific germline MM mutations. Because risk heterogeneity occurs even among carriers of known familial MM genes, such as *CDKN2A*, other unknown genetic variants are thought to also be involved in the development of MM. According to the Melanoma Genetics Consortium, testing for mutations in genes known to be associated with MM should be almost exclusively restricted to research laboratories owing to the unknown penetrance of these mutations, the probable existence of unidentified mutations, and limited data related to prevention and surveillance. It is recommended that clinical testing for specific genetic mutations be reserved for patients with personal or family history of MM, but only when patients can participate in a genetic counseling program. Some families require special attention and consideration for further counseling based on risk alone.

## Associated Diseases

Increased incidence of various other cancers associated with MM and FAMMM syndromes has been described (**Table 18-3**). For example, MM has been reported to account for approximately 7% of all second primary cancers that occur among retinoblastoma patients as well as their kindreds. Atypical nevi are also associated with this group. Pancreatic carcinoma has been positively linked to familial MM, especially in the presence of *CDKN2A* mutations.

**Table 18-3   Pertinent Personal History Predictive of Risk for Malignant Melanoma**

Malignant melanoma

Dysplastic nevi

Freckles in childhood

Ultraviolet light exposure

Multiple sunburns

Pancreatic cancer

Xeroderma pigmentosa

Li-Fraumeni syndrome

Werner's syndrome

Retinoblastoma

More specifically, it has been shown that MM, multiple nevi, and pancreatic carcinoma are inherited as autosomal dominant traits in some MM-affected families. Ocular MM has also been shown to have a correlation with atypical nevi and cutaneous MM within high-risk families. Breast cancer has been reported in association with MM especially among *BRCA1* and *BRCA2* mutation carriers. Other non-melanoma skin cancers, particularly squamous cell carcinoma, and cancers of the nervous system such as neuroblastoma show an association with MM-affected families who exhibit *CDKN2A* mutations.

Clinically, it is important to note the differences between familial melanoma versus melanoma that occurs sporadically. Patients with familial patterns of melanoma tend to be younger at the time of diagnosis (before the age of 30 years) and have more affected first- and second-degree relatives. They are also at greater risk for developing subsequent primary tumors. These high-risk families are significantly more likely to have a poor ability to tan, fair skin color, red hair, and many melanocytic nevi. There appears to be no significant overall difference between high-risk families and other families in terms of the frequency of primary lesion sites, age at the time of diagnosis, distribution of metastases, or survival following diagnosis of MM.

## Management and Treatment

Factors affecting prognosis and treatment of MM include the stage of disease, level of invasion of the primary lesion, location and size of the primary lesion, and general health of the affected person. Management of melanoma includes increased surveillance for the development of new cutaneous lesions as well as metastases. Treatment options depend on the staging results.

Treatment of stage I melanoma involves surgical removal of both the lesion and a margin of unaffected skin. The amount of unaffected skin removed depends on the thickness of the melanoma. No more than 2 cm of normal skin needs to be removed from all sides of stage I melanoma, as wider margins have not been found to improve overall survival. Standard treatment of stage II melanoma comprises wide excision of skin around the tumor site. Sentinel lymph node biopsy is optional at this stage because deeper tumors have an increased risk of spreading to a lymph node.

Stage III melanoma requires the same surgical treatment of the primary lesion as accorded to stage II melanoma, along with lymph node dissection. Adjuvant therapy with α-interferon has been shown to increase disease-free survival in some patients, but has little effect on overall survival. Clinical trials are also an option at this stage.

Stage IV melanoma has a very poor prognosis, given that melanoma cells have spread to distant areas of the body at this stage. Surgery may be performed to debulk the tumors and relieve symptoms depending on the location. Metastases that cannot be removed may be treated with radiation or chemotherapy. Chemotherapy drugs such as dacarbazine and temozolomide can be used, either by themselves or in combination with other drugs, to shrink tumors and slow disease progression. In general, their use does not improve overall survival. Recurrence of melanoma (**recurrent melanoma**) after initial diagnosis is not uncommon regardless of staging.

Moderation—if not outright avoidance—of sun exposure and skin self-examinations (SSE) of nevi are recommended for relatives of affected patients at high risk for developing MM. Melanoma risk is also more highly associated with UV radiation that is intermittent and intense. These factors emphasize the point that patient education is the key to developing a prevention strategy among those deemed at risk for developing this disease.

There is no consensus in the dermatology community regarding surveillance and screening recommendations for relatives of MM patients in high-risk categories. While some investigators recommend that family members of MM patients have any pigmented lesions evaluated, others recommend annual screening of first- and second-degree relatives beginning between 10 and 12 years of age. Specifically, these annual evaluations should include full-body photography, close-up photographs of any atypical nevi, and patient education for SSE; they should be continued at 6-month intervals until nevi are deemed to be stable and the patient is judged to be competent in SSE. Remaining follow-up visits should occur annually thereafter at which time the pedigree should be revised.

Patients who report a personal or family history of ocular melanoma, especially in conjunction with atypical nevi, should be screened for ocular and cutaneous MM. The correlation between *CDKN2A* mutations in MM-affected patients and the development of pancreatic cancer is strong enough to warrant routine surveillance. In members of high-risk families, it is recommended that endoscopic ultrasonography be performed annually beginning at age 50 or 10 years earlier than the age of the youngest relative diagnosed with pancreatic cancer. For individuals who develop **head and neck squamous cell carcinoma** at a young age, annual screening is recommended for pancreatic carcinoma and melanoma.

Currently, there remains a need for established criteria that would define the patient populations at greatest risk and outline specific surveillance plans. Until genetic testing is more readily available and interpretive criteria are established, it is prudent to evaluate all members of families with an excessive number of melanoma cases. For healthcare providers, this care will require paying special attention to the family history to identify patterns of cancer within families and subsequent referral to medical geneticists.

## Chapter Summary

- No single relationship between risk factors and the development of malignant melanoma has been identified, regardless of family history.

- Malignant melanoma is complex in etiology, with multiple pathways being involved in melanomagenesis.

- Diagnosis of familial malignant melanoma requires either two first-degree relatives with malignant melanoma or three relatives of any degree with the disease.

- An accurate family history is the most reliable indicator of risk for development of malignant melanoma, regardless of mutation status.

- Familial atypical multiple mole and melanoma syndrome involves the coexistence of familial malignant melanoma and atypical nevi within families.

- High-risk patients and their families should be counseled on the importance of prevention and surveillance measures such as avoidance of sun exposure, skin self-examinations, and routine follow-up with a dermatologist.

## Key Terms

**Computed tomography (CT) scan:** an imaging procedure that makes a series of detailed pictures of areas inside the body, taken from different angles by using a computer linked to an x-ray machine.

**Covariates:** the interplay of environmental factors with genetic predisposition.

**Head and neck squamous cell carcinoma:** cancer originating from the mucosal lining (epithelium) of the head and neck.

**Lymph node mapping:** a procedure in which a radioactive substance or blue dye is injected near the tumor, then flows through lymph ducts to the first lymph node or nodes where cancer cells are likely to have spread. Lymph nodes that are marked with the dye are then surgically removed and examined microscopically by a pathologist for evidence of cancer cells.

**Magnetic resonance imaging (MRI):** a procedure that uses a magnet, radio waves, and a computer to make a series of detailed images of areas inside the body.

**Melanomagenesis:** the formation of melanoma.

**Penetrance:** the proportion of individuals carrying a particular mutation who express an associated, observable trait.

**Phototype:** a classification system based on a person's sensitivity to sunlight as measured by the ability to tan.

**Positron emission tomography (PET) scan:** an imaging procedure used to locate malignant tumor cells in the body by identifying areas of tissue with greatest glucose utilization.

**Recurrent melanoma:** cancer that has returned after it has been treated to either the original site or in other areas of the body.

**Satellite moles:** new moles that grow in a pattern around existing moles.

**Sentinel node:** the first lymph node to receive lymphatic drainage from a tumor.

**Variable expressivity:** variation in disease symptoms among persons with the same mutation.

**Wide local excision:** a surgical procedure to remove some of the normal tissue surrounding the area where melanoma was found to check for cancer cells not visible on gross examination.

## Chapter Review Questions

1. The single greatest indicator of risk for malignant melanoma is _____.
2. Patients exhibiting familial malignant melanoma are often clinically distinguished from those patients with sporadic malignant melanoma because they are at a _____ age at the time of diagnosis.

3. Which factor confers the highest risk among patients who have a personal history of melanoma? _____.

4. Three important preventive measures for patients at high risk of malignant melanoma are _____, _____, and _____.

5. Other cancers associated with familial melanoma include _____, _____, _____, and _____.

## Resources

Bishop JN, Harland M, Randerson-Moor J, Bishop DT. Management of Familial Melanoma. *Lancet Oncology*. 8(1):46–54; 2007.

Gene Reviews. www.genetests.org.

Genetics Home Reference. http://ghr.nlm.nih.gov/.

Gunder LM. Update on Familial Melanoma: Understanding Risk, Surveillance and the Role of Genetic Testing. *Journal of Dermatology for Physician Assistants*. 2(2):16–21; 2008.

National Cancer Institute, U.S. National Institutes of Health. Breast Cancer Treatment (PDQ®). Available at: http://www.cancer.gov/cancertopics/pdq/treatment/breast/Patient/page5#Keypoint25. Accessed January 27, 2010.

National Cancer Institute, U.S. National Institutes of Health. Melanoma Treatment (PDQ®). Available at: http://www.cancer.gov/cancertopics/pdq/ treatment/melanoma/Patient/print. Accessed January 27, 2010.

Pho L, Grossman D, Leachman SA. Melanoma Genetics: A Review of Genetic Factors and Clinical Phenotypes in Familial Melanoma. *Current Opinions in Oncology*. 18(2):173–179; 2006.

# Chapter 19

# Pharmacogenomics

## CHAPTER OBJECTIVES

✓ Define pharmacogenomics.
✓ Detail some of the challenges associated with drug therapy.
✓ Review example applications of pharmacogenomics.
✓ Identify limitations and pitfalls to this developing technology.

Every practicing clinician has noticed differences among patients in terms of how they react to medicines. This includes not only prescription medications, but also over-the-counter medications (i.e., those obtained without a prescription). Unfortunately, the only way to determine how a patient will react to a medication is via trial and error. Generally, a patient will try some new medicine and then report some adverse reaction soon after starting the treatment. The range of potential reactions varies from some mild itchy skin rash to a full-blown anaphylactic reaction that includes lip and tongue swelling and closing of the airway. Obviously, all healthcare providers want to avoid these types of adverse events in their patients.

**Pharmacogenomics** is the study of how genes affect a person's response to drugs. A relatively new field, it combines pharmacology and genomics to develop effective and safe medications so that doses can be tailored to a person's genetic makeup (Genetics Home Reference, 2010). Along the way, it attempts to explain variability of drug responses based on genetic differences between individuals. The goal is to understand the role that an individual's genetic makeup plays in how well a medicine works, as well as which side effects are likely to occur in the individual's body. This information can help tailor the development of drugs so that they are best suited for a particular individual or group. **Pharmacogenetics** refers to the role of inheritance in individual variation in drug metabolism. For most purposes, the terms "pharmacogenetics" and "pharmacogenomics" can be used interchangeably. Some potential benefits of pharmacogenomics are shown in **Table 19-1**.

Many drugs are altered by enzymes during their metabolism within the body. In some cases, an active drug may be made inactive or less active through metabolism. In other cases, an inactive or less active drug may be made more active through metabolism. The challenge in drug therapy is to make sure that the active form of a drug stays around long enough to do its job: Some people have enzymes that may metabolize a drug too quickly, too slowly, or not at all. Therefore, depending on the situation, the drug may be completely metabolized before it has its intended effect or metabolized very little, leading to unsafe concentrations within the body.

Table 19-1  **Potential Benefits of Pharmacogenomics**

More accurate methods of determining drug dosages

Development of drugs that maximize therapeutic effects but decrease damage to nearby healthy cells

Drug prescribing based on a patient's genetic profile rather than by trial and error; decreased occurrence of adverse reactions

Vaccine development using genetic material, which could activate the immune system similar to current vaccines but with reduced risks of infections

*Source:* Adapted from Barlow-Stewart K, Saleh M. Updated June 2007. Pharmacogenomics/Pharmacogenomics. In: *The Center for Genetics Education* (online). Available at http://www.genetics.com.au/factsheet/fs25.html. Accessed January 18, 2010.

Many currently available drugs are marketed as "one size fits all" therapies, even though they do not work the same way for everyone. It can be difficult to predict who will benefit from a medication, who will not respond at all, and who will experience negative side effects. Unfortunately, adverse drug reactions are a significant cause of hospitalizations and deaths in the United States. Knowledge gained from the Human Genome Project is being used to determine how inherited differences in genes affect the body's response to medications. In the future, these genetic differences may be used to predict whether a medication will be effective for a particular person and to help prevent adverse drug reactions.

The small differences in the genes between different population groups or some families within a population group that have built up over the course of many generations can mean that they react differently to medicines. For example, if one group of people break down a medicine very quickly or very slowly compared to others, then their genes may offer a clue as to why they respond that way. If so, then it may be predicted, based on his or her genes, how someone would react to a medicine prior to giving it.

It is clear that many non-genetic factors (e.g., age, organ function, drug interactions) influence the effects of medications. Nevertheless, genetic variation may account for as much as 95% of variability in some drugs' disposition and effects. There are numerous examples of interindividual differences in drug response caused by common genetic variations (called **polymorphisms**) in genes encoding drug-metabolizing enzymes, drug transporters, or drug targets.

The human genes involved in many pharmacogenetic traits have been identified, and polymorphisms within these genes are in various stages of being exploited as molecular diagnostics in medicine. At present, clinical applications are mostly limited to medications with narrow therapeutic indices (e.g., anticancer agents, some antidepressants, warfarin).

## Drug Metabolism

Several different types of liver enzymes are involved in the metabolism of medications. Genetic variations in these enzymes that affect metabolic rate are relatively common, but the prevalence of the variations differs significantly by ethnic background. Among these enzymes are the cytochrome P450 family (CYP), *N*-acetyltransferase, thiopurine methyl-transferase (TPMT), and UDP-glucuronosyltransferase.

The CYP enzymes include approximately 50 liver enzymes that metabolize more than 30 classes of drugs, including antidepressants, antiepileptics, and cardiovascular drugs. Based on variations in the associated CYP gene, patients can be separated into poor, normal, and ultra-rapid drug metabolizers. Unfortunately, a significant proportion of the population falls into the poor or ultra-rapid metabolizer category. When a patient who is a poor metabolizer of a particular drug is given a standard dose, he or she will process the drug more slowly than expected, resulting in increased levels of the drug in the person's bloodstream. Consequently, there is increased risk for side effects and toxicity. In the case of an ultra-rapid metabolizer, the same dose may be ineffective because the drug is metabolized too rapidly to achieve its maximal effects. Therefore, dosages of these drugs must be modified to accommodate the rate of metabolism.

*N*-Acetyltransferase is a liver enzyme that activates some drugs and deactivates others. Some patients can acetylate (a type of metabolic change) drugs slowly, whereas others acetylate drugs quickly. Those persons who are slow acetylators may experience toxicity when taking drugs such as procainamide, isoniazid, hydralazine, and sulfonamides, whereas those who are fast acetylators may not respond to isoniazid or hydralazine. Between 40% and 70% of Caucasians and African-Americans are considered to be slow acetylators.

Azathioprine and other thiopurine medications (such as 6-mercaptopurine and 6-thioguanine) are used to treat children afflicted with acute lymphocytic leukemia; they are also used to treat inflammatory bowel disease, rheumatoid arthritis, and transplant immune suppression. These immune suppressants are metabolized by TPMT. Because each copy of the TPMT gene will produce some TPMT enzyme, three different groups of enzyme activity levels are distinguished: deficient, intermediate, and normal. Approximately 1 in 300 (0.33%) Caucasians and African Americans are TPMT deficient. Therefore, if these patients are given a standard drug dose, they may suffer severe hematopoietic toxicity. These individuals are able to achieve the desired therapeutic effect from a dose that is one tenth of the recommended dose.

UDP-Glucuronosyltransferase is involved in the metabolism of irinotecan, a chemotherapeutic drug that is used in the treatment of metastatic colorectal cancer. Variations in the gene that codes for this enzyme can influence the patient's ability to break down the major active metabolite in irinotecan. The inability to degrade the metabolite can lead to increased blood concentrations and increased risk of side effects, including reduced white blood cell count and severe diarrhea.

## Warfarin

Warfarin is used to prevent dangerous blood clots from forming in the blood vessels of certain patients, but it can significantly increase the risk of bleeding into the brain or gastrointestinal tract. It is widely known that many clinical and demographic factors, such as age, sex, drug interactions, and diet, affect warfarin's metabolism. In addition, strong evidence indicates that genetic variation contributes to interindividual variability in warfarin's metabolism. Warfarin is primarily metabolized by the cytochrome CYP2C9 enzyme and acts by inhibiting vitamin K epoxide reductase complex subunit 1 (VKORC1). Any genetic variation in the gene sequence coding for both of these enzymes can potentially vary the efficacy and toxicity of warfarin treatment.

The CYP2C9 gene has been linked to toxicity and altered dosage requirements, despite clinicians' ability to titrate warfarin dosing to a clear, effective endpoint (i.e., **International Normalized Ratio** [INR]). For example, in the best-case scenario, a person taking warfarin might maintain a **prothrombin time** of 2 to 3 INR. Patients with a variant CYP2C9 genotype take a median of 95 days longer to achieve stable dosing compared with patients who have a wild-type genotype, however. They also have a higher risk of acute bleeding complications. Patients with the two most common variant alleles require 15% to 30% lower maintenance doses of warfarin to achieve the target INR. When added to clinical factors that are known to affect warfarin dosing, the CYP2C9 genotype has been shown to incrementally improve prediction of warfarin dose maintenance.

Clearly, understanding clinical as well as genetic factors has the potential to improve warfarin therapy. Clinical and demographic variables account for approximately 20% of interindividual variability in warfarin dosing, while the CYP2C9 genotype accounts for 15% to 20% of this variability, and the VKORC1 genotype accounts for an additional 14%. Collectively, 50% to 60% of the total variation in warfarin dosing is predictable before administration—which is very valuable information to the prescribing clinician.

## Cytochrome P450 2D6

Probably the most extensively studied polymorphic drug-metabolizing liver enzyme in humans is cytochrome P450 2D6 (CYP2D6). More than 30 medications are metabolized by this enzyme, including analgesics, antidepressants, and antiemetics. Polymorphisms in the CYP2D6 genotype can cause exaggerated or diminished drug effects, depending on whether the medication is inactivated (e.g., nortriptyline, fluoxetine, 5-hydroxytryptamine inhibitors) or activated (e.g., codeine).

For example, approximately 10% of patients will receive no pain relief from codeine because of the absence of a functional CYP2D6 enzyme, which is responsible for producing the active agent from the **prodrug**. Notably, people with an Asian, Caucasian, or Middle Eastern heritage are less likely to convert codeine into its active morphine form. In contrast, some women are ultra-rapid metabolizers of codeine and are warned against taking the drug during pregnancy or lactation. Consequently, it has been suggested that poor or ultra-rapid metabolizers should not be prescribed this particular agent.

# Pharmacogenomic Tests

Because enzymes involved in drug metabolism arise from multiple genes, pharmacogenomic test results can be difficult to interpret. These test results constitute predictions based on information about the specific genetic variations and on information about the associated diseases, adverse drug reactions, and patient outcomes that have been gathered during studies and clinical trials. In many cases, the predictions will be very accurate, but

Table 19-2  **Some Currently Available Pharmacogenomic Tests**

| Test | Purpose |
|---|---|
| DNA microarray that tests for 29 *CYP2D6* genetic variants and 2 *CYP2C19* genetic variants | Meant to be used as an aid in individualizing treatment selection and dosing for drugs metabolized through these genes. Helps predict poor, intermediate, extensive, or ultra-rapid metabolizers. |
| A test that detects variations in the *UGT1A1* gene, which produces the enzyme UDP-glucuronosyltransferase | Used to identify patients who may be at increased risk of adverse reaction to irinotecan. |
| Tests that detect genetic variants of the CYP2C9 and VKORC1 (vitamin K epoxide reductase) enzymes. | Used to identify patients who have genetic variations and need a reduced dose of warfarin to avoid bleeding episodes. |

*Source:* Data from Pharmacogenomics: Predicting Which Drugs Will Work and Which Won't. Lab Tests Online. Available at http://www.labtestsonline.org/understanding/features/pharmagogenomics -3.html. Accessed January 18, 2010

physicians cannot use the information to state with absolute certainty what will happen with an individual patient. Furthermore, these test results do not incorporate or make allowances for other factors in a patient's life related to the disease condition or to the individual that may affect the response to treatment. Therefore, the results are intended to be used in conjunction with other relevant clinical findings.

Some currently available pharmacogenomic tests are shown in **Table 19-2**. In 2005, a Food and Drug Administration advisory committee voted in favor of changing warfarin's label to reflect the fact that pharmacogenomic information can be useful in deciding a patient's individual dose.

## Limitations and Ethical Issues

Because many genes are likely to play at least some role in how someone reacts to a drug, the idea of targeting different drugs represents a very complex challenge (**Table 19-3**). Another consideration is that interactions with other drugs and environmental factors may influence a specific drug reaction. Consequently, the influence of these factors will need to be elucidated before conclusions are drawn about how a specific drug is working.

While the idea of individually targeted drug therapy is very attractive, it is likely to be very expensive—a consideration that will affect the access to such drugs for many people. Of course, there is always the issue of whether health insurance plans will cover the cost. Given these factors, the future of pharmacogenomics will most likely focus on the development of drugs that work well with certain population groups. However, any program will need to be carefully implemented to avoid a perception of stigma based on ethnicity.

**Table 19-3   Limitations to Taking Full Advantage of Pharmacogenomics**

Many genes are likely involved in how someone reacts to a drug, making targeted drugs very complex.

Identification of the small variations in everyone's genes that may influence drug metabolism or how the condition develops is very difficult and time consuming.

Interactions with other drugs and environmental factors will need to be determined before any conclusions are reached about genetic influence on how the drug is working.

*Source:* Adapted from Barlow-Stewart K, Saleh M. Updated June 2007. Pharmacogenomics/Pharmacogenomics. In: *The Center for Genetics Education* (online). Available at http://www.genetics.com.au/factsheet/fs25.html. Accessed January 18, 2010.

Because not all people who belong to a particular ethnic group will have the same genetic variations, the assumption that an individual's race can indicate his or her genetic profile for drug response can be a potential problem. A possible consequence of such genetic profiling is denial of treatment based on race if a pharmacogenomic test is not available for a particular drug. Thus people from different ethnic groups who are affected by the same condition may be given different access to treatment.

## Chapter Summary

- Pharmacogenomics combines pharmacology and genomics to develop effective and safe medications so that doses can be tailored to a person's genetic makeup.

- Many currently available drugs are marketed as "one size fits all" options, even though they do not work the same way for everyone.

- Adverse drug reactions are a significant cause of hospitalizations and deaths in the United States.

- Pharmacogenomic test results are predictions based on information about the specific genetic variations and on information about the associated diseases, adverse drug reactions, and patient outcomes that have been gathered during studies and clinical trials.

- While the idea of individually targeted drug therapy is very attractive, it is likely to be very expensive, a factor that will affect the accessibility of such drugs for many people.

## Key Terms

**International Normalized Ratio (INR):** a system established by the World Health Organization and the International Committee on Thrombosis and Hemostasis for reporting the results of blood coagulation (clotting) tests. All results are standardized using the international sensitivity index for the particular thromboplastin reagent and instrument combination used to perform the test. No matter which laboratory checks the prothrombin time, the result should be the same even if different thromboplastins and instruments are used.

**Pharmacogenetics:** the study of the interrelation of hereditary constitution and response to drugs.

**Pharmacogenomics:** the combination of pharmacology and genomics in an effort to develop effective and safe medications in a way that compensates for genetic differences in patients that cause varied responses to a single therapeutic regimen.

**Polymorphisms:** natural variations in a gene, DNA sequence, or chromosome that have no adverse effects on the individual and occur with fairly high frequency in the general population.

**Prodrug:** a class of drugs in which the pharmacologic action results from conversion by metabolic processes within the body.

**Prothrombin time:** a clotting test done to test the integrity of part of the clotting scheme, which is commonly used as a method of monitoring the accuracy of blood thinning treatment (anticoagulation) with warfarin. The test measures the time needed for clot formation after thromboplastin (plus calcium) has been added to plasma.

## Chapter Review Questions

1. Pharmacogenomics attempts to explain variability of drug responses based on _____ between individuals.

2. Many drugs are altered by _____ during metabolism in the body.

3. Genetic variation can account for as much as _____ of variability in drug disposition and effects.

4. Approximately 50 liver cytochrome P450 enzymes metabolize more than 30 classes of drugs, including _____, _____, and _____.

5. Many clinical and demographic factors, such as _____, _____, _____, and _____, affect warfarin dosing.

## Resources

A list of clinical trials involving pharmacogenomics is available at ClinicalTrials.gov (http://clinicaltrials.gov/ct2/results?term=pharmacogenomics).

Genetics Home Reference. What Is Pharmacogenomics? Available at: http://ghr.nlm .nih.gov/handbook/genomicresearch/pharmacogenomics. Accessed January 27, 2010.

Kalow W, Meyer UA, Tyndale R. *Pharmacogenomics.* New York: CRC Press; 2001.

Lanfear DE, McLeod HL. Pharmacogenetics: Using DNA to Optimize Drug Therapy. *American Family Physician.* 76:1179–1182; 2007.

Massachusetts Pain Initiative. http://www.masspaininitiative.org/PDFs/Pain%20 Facts%20Sept%202008.pdf.

Medicinenet.com. http://www.medterms.com/script/main/hp.asp.

*Merriam-Webster Online.* http://www.merriam-webster.com/.

National Center for Biotechnology Information. http://www.ncbi.nlm.nih.gov/ About/primer/pharm.html.

National Institute of General Medical Sciences. http://www.nigms.nih.gov/Initia tives/PGRN/Background/pgrn_faq.htm.

Personalized Healthcare Report 2008: Warfarin and Genetic Testing. http://www .ama-assn.org/ama1/pub/upload/mm/464/warfarin_brochure.pdf.

Pharmacogenetics/Pharmacogenomics: Fact Sheet 25. Centre for Genetics Education. http://www.genetics.com.au/pdf/factsheets/fs25.pdf.

Pharmacogenomics: Human Genome Project Information. http://www.ornl.gov/ sci/techresources/ Human_ Genome/medicine/pharma.shtml.

Pharmacogenomics: Lab Tests Online. http://www.labtestsonline.org/understand ing/features/pharmacogenomics.html.

*Stedman's Online Medical Dictionary.* www.stedmans.com.

Westman JA. *Medical Genetics for the Modern Clinician.* Philadelphia: Lippincott Williams & Wilkins; 2006.

# Chapter 20

# Gene Therapy

## CHAPTER OBJECTIVES

✓ Describe the basic principles of gene therapy.
✓ Identify the various types of gene therapy.
✓ Detail how various viruses are used as delivery vehicles for new
   genetic information.
✓ Review the problems and pitfalls associated with gene therapy.

Given the exciting genetic progress that has been made over the past few years such as through the Human Genome Project, it is natural to speculate how this new information might be used to address various human genetic diseases. On an almost daily basis, an announcement is released to the media that another important gene involved in some disease has been identified. Thus it might seem that the concept of taking out the "bad" gene and replacing it with a "good" gene would lend itself to rather straightforward application. In fact, the basic premise of gene therapy is to insert a "normal" gene into the genome to replace an "abnormal" disease-causing gene. Even though this sounds simple, in reality it is very challenging.

Some approaches currently under investigation include using gene therapy for the following purposes:

- Exchange an abnormal gene for a normal gene through homologous recombination

- Repair an abnormal gene through selective reverse mutation, which returns the gene to its normal function

- Alter the regulation (the degree to which a gene is turned on or off) of a particular gene

## Basic Process

Because adding naked DNA or RNA to a cell is an inefficient process, most gene therapy uses some type of gene delivery vehicle. A carrier molecule called a **vector** is frequently used to deliver the therapeutic gene to the patient's target cells. Currently, the most common vector is a virus that has been genetically altered to carry normal human DNA. Viruses have evolved a way of encapsulating and delivering their genes to human cells in a pathogenic manner. Researchers have tried to take advantage of this capability and manipulate the virus genome so as to remove disease-causing genes and insert therapeutic genes.

Gene transfer strategies involve three essential elements: (1) a vector, (2) a gene to be delivered, and (3) a relevant target cell to which the DNA or RNA is delivered. Gene delivery

Table 20-1 **Breakdown of Clinical Gene Transfer Studies by Disease Classification**

| Disease | Percentage |
|---|---|
| Cancer | 64.5% |
| Vascular diseases | 8.7% |
| Monogenic diseases | 8.2% |
| Infectious diseases | 8.0% |
| Other diseases | 2.4% |
| Gene marking | 3.0% |
| Healthy volunteers | 2.3% |

*Source:* Gene Therapy Clinical Trials Worldwide. *Journal of Gene Medicine.* 2010. http://www.abedia.com/wiley/indications.php. Accessed August 13, 2010.

can take place in vivo, in which the vector is directly injected into the patient, or, in the case of hematopoietic and some other target cells, ex vivo, in which the target cells are removed from the patient, followed by return of the modified autologous cells after gene transfer in the laboratory. When the donated DNA enters the target cell and begins expression, this process is referred to as **transduction**.

Gene therapy is far from being characterized as a routine treatment regimen at this point. In fact, it is one of the most complex therapeutic modalities yet attempted, and each new disease represents a therapeutic problem for which dosing, safety, and efficacy must be defined. Nevertheless, gene transfer remains one of the most powerful and promising concepts in modern molecular medicine: It has the potential to address a host of diseases for which there are currently no cures or, in some cases, no available treatment. More than 6000 subjects have been enrolled in gene transfer studies to date, and serious adverse events have been rare. As outlined in **Table 20-1**, gene therapies are being developed for a wide variety of disease processes, although the majority of trials so far have addressed cancer, with cardiovascular diseases and monogenic disorders representing the next most popular categories.

## Types of Gene Therapy

In theory, it is possible to transform either somatic cells (most cells of the body) or cells of the germline (such as sperm cells, ova, and their stem cell precursors). Historically, gene therapy in people has historically been directed at somatic cells, whereas germline modification in humans remains highly controversial. Not all somatic cells are good candidates for gene therapy. Specifically, good candidates should be easily accessible and have a long life span within the body. Proliferating cells are preferred for some gene delivery systems because the vector carrying the gene of interest can integrate itself into the replicating DNA of the cell. While bone marrow stem cells meet all of these requirements, they are difficult to manipulate as well as to isolate from bone marrow. Therefore, a variety of other cell types are being investigated as potential targets, including skin fibroblasts, muscle cells, vascular endothelial cells, hepatocytes, and lymphocytes.

Most current gene therapy approaches involve the replacement of a missing gene product by insertion of a normal gene into a somatic cell to correct **loss-of-function mutations**. These types of mutations result in a nonfunctional or missing gene product; insertion of the normal gene corrects this defect. Potentially, many recessive disorders may be corrected with the production of only a small amount of the gene product.

## Viruses as Gene Therapy Vectors

Many techniques have been developed for introducing genes into different cell types, although not all are applicable or feasible in somatic cells. Because viruses have evolved ways to insert their genes into cells with high efficiency, they have received a lot of focus as potential gene therapy vectors. As described in this section, several types of viruses are being investigated, with varying degrees of success. Note that these viral vectors have been modified using molecular techniques to prevent replication and subsequent infection of the host.

### Retroviruses

A retrovirus can create double-stranded DNA copies of its RNA genome, which can then be integrated into the chromosomes of host cells. Such viruses become integrated into the host DNA with a high degree of efficiency and seldom induce an immune response. Because these modified retroviruses are unable to replicate, they are propagated in **packaging cells**, which allows for production of multiple copies that contain the human gene but cannot replicate themselves (**Figure 20-1**). The modified retroviruses are then incubated with the

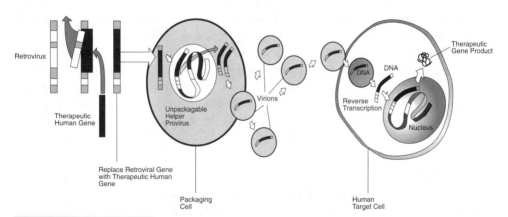

**Figure 20-1** Use of a retroviral vector for gene therapy. Replication of the retrovirus is prevented by removing most of its genome; a normal human gene is then inserted into the retrovirus and propagated in a packaging cell. Virions from the packaging cell are incubated with human somatic cells, which allow the retrovirus to insert copies of the normal human gene into the cell. Once integrated into the cell's DNA, the inserted gene produces normal gene product. *Source:* Reproduced with permission from Jorde LB, Carey JC, Bamshad MJ, White RL. *Medical Genetics*, 3rd ed. 2006.

somatic cells (e.g., bone marrow stem cells) obtained from a patient and the modified retrovirus inserts the normal human gene into the host cell. Once inserted, the normal gene will encode for a normal gene product in the patient's somatic cells. This approach has been used to treat many diseases, including **severe combined immune deficiency**.

Even though there are advantages to using retroviruses as vectors in gene therapy, this approach also has certain disadvantages. One important concern relates to their potential to induce tumor formation. Because a retrovirus becomes integrated into gene-rich regions of the host's DNA, it could activate a nearby **proto-oncogene**, resulting in tumor formation. Another disadvantage is that retroviruses infect only dividing cells; they are ineffective in nondividing or slowly dividing cells such as neurons. Of course, if the goal is to target only dividing cells, then this limitation may actually be beneficial. One example would be in the treatment of a brain tumor where the **neoplastic** cells are dividing but the nearby brain cells are not.

## Adenoviruses

**Adenoviruses** contain double-stranded DNA. This class of viruses causes respiratory, intestinal, and eye infections in humans, including the common cold. Prior to their use as a gene therapy vector, adenoviruses must be modified so that they are unable to replicate. They are able to infect both dividing and nondividing cells, but do not become integrated into the host cell's genome. Thus gene expression following adenoviral gene transfer is short-lived. However, because these viruses do not become integrated into the genome of the host, they will not activate a proto-oncogene, as might occur with a retrovirus. Based on their ability to infect nondividing cells, adenoviruses are being used in trials to deliver the normal **CFTR gene** to lung epithelial cells by an aerosol. Researchers hope that this novel approach will increase chloride-ion channel activity in patients with cystic fibrosis (see Chapter 11).

One disadvantage of their short life span is that eventually these adenoviruses will become inactivated and will then need to be readministered for therapeutic purposes. Another problem is that typically only part of the adenovirus genome is removed, which can lead to stimulation of the host's immune response. This problem increases with repeated adenovirus exposure as the foreign protein further stimulates the immune response. Researchers are attempting to remove more of the viral genome in an effort to reduce the immune response.

## Adeno-associated Viruses

Parvovirus is an example of an **adeno-associated virus**—one of a class of small, single-stranded DNA viruses that can insert their genetic material at a specific site on chromosome 19. **Fifth disease** is caused by infection with human parvovirus B19 and infects only humans. It manifests as a mild rash illness that occurs most commonly in children. While adeno-associated viruses are smaller than either retroviruses or adenoviruses, they have the advantage that they stimulate little, if any, immune response from the host and can enter nondividing cells.

As discussed in Chapter 8, hemophilia is caused by a deficiency of either factor VIII (hemophilia A) or factor IX (hemophilia B) and can require lifelong therapy. In early experiments with gene therapy to treat this condition, researchers injected an adeno-associated virus with the factor IX gene into the skeletal muscle of mice, which resulted in the production of sustained levels of this factor above the therapeutic range. More recently, similar experiments have been carried out in several human patients with hemophilia B. In one individual, the treatment resulted in sustained expression of factor IX at 1% of the normal level. While this response is insufficient to cure this disease, this low level of expression significantly reduced the number of factor IX treatments needed to control bleeding.

## Other Viral Sources

**Herpes simplex viruses** are a class of double-stranded DNA viruses that infect a particular cell type, specifically the neurons. Herpes simplex virus type 1 is a common human pathogen that causes cold sores, whereas herpes simplex virus type 2 is associated with genital lesions. This vector is being investigated in an attempt to take advantage of its ability to insert DNA into frequently inaccessible neurons.

In addition to simple retroviruses, complex retroviruses known as **lentiviruses** also exist that can enter nondividing cells through pores in the nuclear membrane. An example of a lentivirus is the human immunodeficiency virus (HIV). These viruses are stably integrated into the genome.

# Challenges Associated with Viral Vectors

While the carrier of choice in most gene therapy studies is some type of virus, use of this approach presents a variety of potential problems to the patient (**Table 20-2**). For example, because only some (not all) of the target cells may successfully incorporate the normal gene, the desired gene product may be expressed at subtherapeutic levels in the host. This result is not necessarily always a negative outcome, however, as transient expression may be adequate in some types of therapy.

As mentioned earlier, it may be difficult to target neurons associated with central nervous system disorders. By comparison, systemic disorders may prove relatively easy to target by modifying lymphocytes or bone marrow stem cells. Nevertheless, there is always the fear that the viral vector, once inside the patient, may recover its ability to cause disease.

**Table 20-2  Potential Pitfalls Associated with Using Viral Gene Therapy**

Transient and low-level expression

Toxicity

Immune and inflammatory response

Difficulty reaching target tissue

Need for precise regulation of gene activity

Potential for mutagenesis

Viral reactivation in host

*Sources:* High KA. Gene Therapy in Clinical Medicine. In Fauci AS, et al. *Harrison's Principles of Internal Medicine.* 2008; Jorde et al. *Medical Genetics,* 3rd ed. 2006.

Whenever a foreign object is introduced into human tissues, the immune system is induced to attack the foreign substance. Therefore, the possibility that the vector might stimulate the immune system in a way that reduces the gene therapy's effectiveness is always a risk. In addition, the immune system's enhanced response to intruders it has seen before makes it difficult for gene therapy to be repeated in patients.

Another pitfall associated with current viral gene therapy is the inability to achieve precise regulation of gene activity. While this factor may not be critical for some diseases, it is critical for diseases such as **thalassemia**, where the number of globin chains must be balanced in a narrow range.

## Alternative Gene Delivery Systems

Besides virus-mediated gene delivery systems, several nonviral options are being explored as means to administer gene therapy. The simplest method involves the direct introduction of therapeutic DNA into target cells. Unfortunately, the main limitation to this approach is that it can be used only with certain tissues and requires large amounts of DNA.

Another nonviral alternative involves the creation of an artificial lipid sphere with an aqueous core or **liposome**. Owing to the lipophilic nature associated with the liposome, the therapeutic DNA would be capable of passing through the target cell's membrane. One advantage of the liposome is that it does not stimulate an immune response because it does not contain any peptides. Conversely, the main disadvantage is that it does not have a transfer efficiency equivalent to that of viruses.

Therapeutic DNA also can get inside target cells by chemically linking the DNA to a molecule that will bind to special cell receptors. Once bound to these receptors, the therapeutic DNA molecules are engulfed by the cell membrane and passed into the interior of the target cell. This delivery system tends to be less effective than other options, however.

An interesting concept that has recently emerged focuses on the use of human artificial chromosomes. These synthetically constructed chromosomes contain functional centromeres and telomeres, so they should be able to integrate and replicate in human cell nuclei. **Table 20-3** summarizes some advantages and disadvantages of several proposed gene delivery vehicles.

While gene replacement techniques are being investigated to correct loss-of-function mutations, these techniques are not adequate to correct gain-of-function or dominant negative mutations (e.g., those causing Marfan syndrome or Huntington's disease). Rather than trying to increase synthesis of a defective gene product, in neutralizing **gain-of-function mutations** the defective gene product must be disabled or prevented from being synthesized. Several gene-blocking methods (antisense therapy, ribozyme therapy, and RNA interference) are being evaluated to see whether they might be effective in alleviating some of these diseases.

Antisense therapy involves the synthesis of an **oligonucleotide** containing DNA that is complementary to that of the messenger RNA sequence produced by a gain-of-function mutation. The binding of this oligonucleotide to the abnormal messenger RNA prevents translation of the harmful protein. This approach is being used to disrupt expression of **oncogenes** involved in pancreatic and colorectal cancers.

Table 20-3  **Advantages and Disadvantages of Gene Delivery Vehicles**

| Vector | Advantage | Disadvantage |
|---|---|---|
| Retroviral | Persistent gene transfer in dividing cells | Theoretical risk of insertional mutagenesis |
| Lentiviral | Persistent gene transfer in transduced tissues | Might induce oncogenesis in some cases |
| Adenoviral | Highly effective in transducing various tissues | Viral capsid elicits strong immune responses |
| Adeno-associated virus | Elicits few inflammatory responses, nonpathogenic | Limited packaging capacity |
| Herpes simplex virus 1 | Large packaging capacity with persistent gene transfer | Residual cytotoxicity with neuron specificity |
| Liposomes | Transfects many cell types; large holding capacity to enable a high number of base pairs | Expensive to produce |
| Naked DNA | Efficient in gene transfer; limited immunogenicity | Transient and low-level expression |

*Source:* Adapted from High KA. Gene Therapy in Clinical Medicine. In Fauci AS, et al. *Harrison's Principles of Internal Medicine.* 17th ed; 2008, pp 420–423.

**Ribozymes** are RNA molecules with enzyme activity that can cleave messenger RNA. As a consequence, they might potentially be engineered to disrupt specific mutation-causing sequences within the messenger RNA molecule before translation occurs. This therapy is being explored as a way to prevent overexpression of certain receptors involved in many breast tumors.

The last type of gene blocking involves RNA interference, a strategy that cells have evolved to defend themselves against viral invasion. Many viruses contain double-stranded RNA. When cells of multicellular organisms detect this type of RNA, an enzyme is induced to digest the foreign RNA by breaking it into small pieces. These pieces are then used as a template to direct the destruction of any single-stranded viral RNA. By artificially synthesizing double-stranded RNA molecules that correspond to a disease-causing DNA sequence, RNA interference might potentially be induced to destroy the messenger RNA produced by a mutated sequence. This approach has shown some promise in reducing transcripts produced by some oncogenes as well as the *bcr/abl* fusion gene associated with chronic myelogenous leukemia (see Chapter 7).

In addition to the limitations detailed previously regarding viral gene therapy, several other factors may prevent gene therapy from becoming an effective treatment for genetic diseases. One goal is to ensure that the therapeutic DNA introduced into target cells remains functional and that the cells containing the therapeutic DNA are long lived and stable. Unfortunately, problems with integrating therapeutic DNA into the genome as well as the rapidly dividing nature of many cells prevent gene therapy from achieving any long-term benefits. Such a short-lived response means that patients will have to undergo multiple rounds of gene therapy.

Disorders that arise from single-gene mutations are currently the best candidates for gene therapy. However, some of the most commonly occurring disorders seen in everyday clinical practice—such as heart disease, high blood pressure, Alzheimer's disease, hyperlipidemia, arthritis, and diabetes—involve the combined effects of many gene variations. Therefore, multigene or multifactorial disorders present another limitation in that they are especially difficult to treat effectively using gene therapy.

## Recent Progress

**Table 20-4** summarizes a few recent developments in the use of gene therapy to address different disease processes in humans, although it is not meant to be an all-inclusive listing. Most gene therapy studies involve only a few patients, so their results usually do not reflect findings from large patient populations. Nevertheless, some of the results are very promising. To obtain more up-to-date information regarding gene therapy clinical trials, the following Web sites are recommended:

- Clinicaltrials.gov: http://clinicaltrials.gov/search/term=gene%2Btherapy
- Gene therapy clinical trials worldwide: http://www.wiley.co.uk/genetherapy/clinical/

Table 20-4   **Examples of Recent Progress in Gene Therapy Research**

| Disease | Gene Therapy | Result |
|---|---|---|
| Leber's congenital amaurosis—a rare inherited eye disease due to mutation in the *RPE65* gene | Recombinant adeno-associated virus vector expressing *RPE65* | Significant improvement in visual function |
| Lung cancer tumors | Gene delivery using lipid-based nanoparticles | Reduction in number and size of tumors in mice |
| Advanced metastatic melanoma | Normal lymphocytes infected with modified retrovirus | Cancer regression and patients who remained disease-free for more than one year |

*Source:* Data from Gene Therapy. Human Genome Project Information. Available at http://www.ornl.gov/sci/techresources/Human_Genome/medicine/genetherapy.shtml#recent. Accessed January 18, 2010.

## Chapter Summary

- The basic premise underlying gene therapy is the insertion of a "normal" gene into the genome to replace an "abnormal," disease-causing gene.

- A carrier molecule called a vector is frequently used to deliver the therapeutic gene to the patient's target cells.
- Because viruses have evolved ways to insert their genes into cells with high efficiency, they have received a great deal of attention as potential gene therapy vectors.
- Gene transfer strategies involve three essential elements: (1) a vector, (2) a gene to be delivered, and (3) a relevant target cell to which the DNA or RNA is delivered.
- Proliferating cells are preferred for some gene delivery systems because the vector carrying the gene of interest can become integrated into the replicating DNA of the cell.
- Gene therapy is far from being characterized as a routine treatment regimen, as it is one of the most complex therapeutic modalities yet attempted. Each new disease represents a therapeutic problem for which dosing, safety, and efficacy must be defined.

## Key Terms

**Adeno-associated virus:** any of a class of small, single-stranded DNA viruses that can insert their genetic material at a specific site on chromosome 19. Parvovirus is an example of this type of virus.

**Adenovirus:** any of a class of viruses that contain double-stranded DNA and cause respiratory, intestinal, and eye infections in humans.

**CFTR gene:** the cystic fibrosis transmembrane conductance regulator gene, which helps create sweat, digestive juices, and mucus. Cystic fibrosis develops because of mutations in this gene.

**Fifth disease:** a disease caused by infection with human parvovirus B19, which infects only humans. It manifests as a mild rash illness that occurs most commonly in children. The ill child typically has a "slapped-cheek" rash on the face and a lacy red rash on the trunk and limbs.

**Gain-of-function mutation:** a mutation that results in a protein product that either is increased in quantity or has a novel function.

**Herpes simplex virus:** any of a class of double-stranded DNA viruses that infect a particular cell type, specifically the neurons.

**Lentivirus:** a type of complex retrovirus that can enter nondividing cells through pores in the nuclear membrane. Human immunodeficiency virus is an example.

**Liposome:** an artificial lipid sphere with an aqueous core.

**Loss-of-function mutation:** a type of mutation that results in a nonfunctional or missing gene product; insertion of the normal gene corrects this defect.

**Neoplastic:** related to the pathologic process that results in the formation and growth of a neoplasm or abnormal tissue that may be either benign or malignant.

**Oligonucleotide:** a DNA sequence consisting of a small number of nucleotide bases.

**Oncogene:** a gene that can transform cells so that they enter into a highly proliferative state that causes cancer.

**Packaging cells:** cells in which replication-deficient viruses are placed so that the replication machinery of the packaging cell can produce viral copies.

**Proto-oncogene:** a gene whose protein product is involved in the regulation of cell growth. When altered, a proto-oncogene can become a cancer-causing oncogene.

**Ribozymes:** RNA molecules with enzyme activity that can cleave messenger RNA.

**Severe combined immune deficiency:** any of a group of rare, sometimes fatal, congenital disorders characterized by little or no immune response.

**Thalassemia:** any of a group of inherited disorders of hemoglobin metabolism in which there is impaired synthesis of one or more of the polypeptide chains of globin.

**Transduction:** transfer of genetic material (and its phenotypic expression) from one cell to another by viral infection.

**Vector:** the vehicle used to carry a DNA insert (e.g., a virus).

## Chapter Review Questions

1. A carrier molecule called a _____ is frequently used to deliver a therapeutic gene to target cells.

2. Gene transfer strategies involve three essential elements: _____, _____, and _____.

3. Most current gene therapy approaches involve the replacement of a missing gene product by inserting a normal gene into a somatic cell to correct _____.

4. The class of viruses whose members contain double-stranded DNA and cause respiratory, intestinal, and eye infections in humans is called _____.

5. In _____, the defective gene product must be disabled or prevented from being synthesized.

## Resources

Castro Januario E, Kipps Thomas J. Principles of Gene Transfer For Therapy. In: Lichtman MA, Beutler E, Kipps TJ, Seligsohn U, Kaushansky K, Prchal JT (Eds.), *Williams Hematology*, 7th ed. http://www.accessmedicine.com/content.aspx?aID =2139222.

Gene Therapy Clinical Trials Worldwide. *Journal of Gene Medicine.* December 2009. http://www.abedia.com/wiley/indications.php.

Gene Therapy: Human Genome Project information. U.S. Department of Energy Office of Science, Office of Biological and Environmental Research, Human Genome Program. http://www.ornl.gov/sci/techresources/Human_Genome/medicine/gene therapy.shtml.

High KA. Gene Therapy in Clinical Medicine. In: Fauci AS, Braunwald E, Kasper DL, Hauser SL, Longo DL, Jameson JL, Loscalzo J (Eds.), *Harrison's Principles of Internal Medicine*, 17th ed. New York: McGraw-Hill Medical; 2008, pp. 420–423.

Jorde LB, Carey JC, Bamshad MJ, White RL. *Medical Genetics,* 3rd ed. St. Louis, MO: Mosby; 2006.

Morgan RA, Dudley ME, Wunderlich JR, Hughes MS, Yang JC, Sherry RM, et al. Cancer Regression in Patients Mediated by Transfer of Genetically Engineered Lymphocytes. *Science Express.* August 31, 2006.

National Cancer Institute, U.S. National Institutes of Health. http://www.cancer .gov/newscenter/pressreleases/MelanomaGeneTherapy.

Parvovirus B19 (Fifth Disease). National Center for Immunization and Respiratory Diseases, Division of Viral Diseases. http://www.cdc.gov/ncidod/dvrd/revb/res piratory/parvo_b19.htm.

Severe Combined Immunodeficiency. Genes and Disease. http://www.ncbi.nlm.nih .gov/books/bv.fcgi?call=bv.View..ShowSection&rid=gnd.section.153.

*Stedman's Online Medical Dictionary.* http://www.stedmans.com/.

Westman JA. *Medical Genetics for the Modern Clinician.* Philadelphia: Lippincott Williams & Wilkins; 2006.

# Chapter 21

# Ethical, Legal, and Social Issues

## CHAPTER OBJECTIVES

✓ Discuss ethical, legal, and social issues related to genetic testing.
✓ Identify factors to discuss with a patient prior to and after genetic testing.
✓ Emphasize that complete confidentiality of genetic test results cannot be guaranteed.
✓ Review bioethics principles that all healthcare providers need to incorporate into their practice.

It is anticipated that in the future, genetic information will play an increasingly larger role in the screening, diagnosis, and treatment of disease. While these advances are intended to improve the health of the population, the potential for negative effects cannot be ignored. This chapter explores the question of how advances in medical genetics might adversely affect patients.

One important negative is the possibility that sensitive genetic information might be used by insurance companies and employers to discriminate against certain individuals. For example, if a person has a chronic long-term disease (i.e., sickle cell anemia, cystic fibrosis), a health insurance company may not want to deal with the economic consequences associated with the medical management of that disease and may refuse to provide coverage for a known genetic predilection. Similarly, if an insurance provider knows that an individual or family has a positive genetic test for hereditary breast and ovarian cancer or familial adenomatous polyposis, the economic consequences to the affected individuals and family members could be devastating if the insurance company denies coverage for that condition.

## Genetic Testing

As genetic testing for disease susceptibility becomes incorporated into clinical practice to a greater extent, primary care providers will increasingly initiate genetic counseling and referrals for testing. However, genetic testing is associated with many ethical, social, and legal concerns that need to be addressed during the counseling process (**Table 21-1**). For example, informed consent requires discussion of the limitations of available genetic tests and interventions, implications of the test results for the patient and family members, and limits of confidentiality as well as discrimination risks posed by such testing. Other issues include regulatory concerns associated with commercial testing and existing legal protections against genetic discrimination.

**Table 21-1  Guidelines for Pre-test Education, Informed Consent, and Post-test Counseling**

1.  Obtain an accurate family history and confirm the diagnosis before testing.

2.  Provide information about the natural history of the condition and the purpose of the test.

3.  Discuss the predictive value of the test, technical accuracy of the test, and meaning of a positive versus negative result.

4.  Explore options for approximation of risk without genetic testing.

5.  Identify the patient's motives for undergoing the test, the potential impact of testing on relatives, and the risk of passing a mutation on to children.

6.  Discuss the potential risk of psychosocial distress to the patient and family even if no mutation is found.

7.  Explain the logistics of testing and the fees involved for testing and counseling.

8.  Discuss issues involving confidentiality and risk of employment and insurance discrimination.

9.  Describe medical options, efficacy of available surveillance and prevention methods, and recommendations for screening if test results are negative.

10.  Provide a written summary of counseling session content.

11.  Obtain informed consent for testing.

12.  Provide test results in person and offer follow-up support.

*Source:* White MT, Callif-Daley F, Donnelly J. Genetic Testing for Disease Susceptibility: Social, Ethical and Legal  Issues for Family Physicians. *American Family Physician.* 60:748, 750, 755, 757–758; 1999.

Genetic testing for mutations that may influence disease susceptibility is appropriate for those relatively few patients who are known to be at high risk. Consequently, testing is not usually suggested until patients, or their family members, have received genetic counseling. Ideally, testing will begin with a living family member who has been diagnosed with a genetic disease. Such testing is performed to determine the presence or absence of a responsible mutation within the individual; this information can then be used to establish or confirm a diagnosis. Unfortunately, many genetic tests do not identify all possible mutations, so test results can be ambiguous in the absence of a known mutation.

Pretest counseling includes risk assessment, discussion of testing alternatives, and the predictive value and interpretive limitations of the test(s). Risk assessment involves taking a detailed family history, with the provider then estimating disease risks associated with specific mutations. Patients need to consider any medical benefits provided by this kind of testing, the psychological implications of the test result, and the significance of testing for family members. Potential benefits of testing typically include relief of anxiety, opportunities for behavior modification, and increased surveillance or interventions that may reduce risk (**Table 21-2**). Negatives include "survivor guilt," increased anxiety, depression,

Table 21-2　**Benefits and Risks Associated with Genetic Testing**

| Benefits | Risks |
| --- | --- |
| Emotional relief and/or reassurance | Psychological stress |
| Provide knowledge that may affect future decisions | Strained family relationships |
| Provide opportunities for increased surveillance or risk-reducing behaviors | Confidentiality/disclosure issues |
| | Insurance and/or employment discrimination |

*Source:* White MT, Callif-Daley F, Donnelly J. Genetic Testing for Disease Susceptibility: Social, Ethical and Legal  Issues for Family Physicians. *American Family Physician.* 60:748, 750, 755, 757–758; 1999.

anger, and the potential for discrimination by insurers and employers. Whether a genetic test is positive or negative, its results have implications for major life decisions.

Post-test counseling ensures that the test results are interpreted correctly. It is important that patients fully understand that a positive test result represents only a probability; it does not necessarily guarantee that they will get that disease. Similarly, a negative test result does not guarantee that a disease will not develop. For example, a woman may receive a negative test result for known breast cancer mutations, but she needs to be educated that she is still at risk for developing breast cancer just like the other women in the general population without known breast cancer mutations.

## Confidentiality

All patients need to be aware that their genetic information may be requested by third parties, including family members, insurers, employers, or other physicians. Prior to undergoing genetic testing, a patient needs to understand that complete confidentiality may be difficult to ensure and that disclosure of genetic information to insurers and employers may have discriminatory consequences. For example, patients could be denied access to health insurance, employment, education, and even loans based on their test results.

The Health Insurance Portability and Accountability Act of 1996 (HIPAA) was designed to provide some protection from discrimination. Unfortunately, HIPAA does not prohibit the use of genetic information as a basis for charging a group more for health insurance, limit the collection of genetic information by insurers, prohibit insurers from requiring an individual to take a genetic test, limit the disclosure of genetic information by insurers, or apply to individual health insurers except if covered by the portability provision.

Many state legislatures have passed laws to govern health insurance and protect the rights to privacy of any individual. In general, these laws define what counts as "genetic information," prohibit insurers from engaging in discriminatory practices based on that information, and require written informed consent by a patient before disclosure of test results to third parties. Unfortunately, the main loophole in the state laws has related to the definition of genetic information, which is usually limited to results of DNA, RNA, or chromosomal analysis. In reality, genetic information may also be obtained from a patient's medical record, family history, and laboratory results to which these laws may not apply. Moreover, in some cases, employer-based group plans are exempt from state regulation.

To overcome the limitations associated with HIPAA and some state laws, a new federal law that prohibits discrimination in health coverage and employment based on genetic information was signed into law on May 21, 2008. The **Genetic Information Nondiscrimination Act of 2008 (GINA)** provides a baseline level of protection against genetic discrimination for all Americans. As mentioned previously, many states already have laws that protect against genetic discrimination in health insurance and employment situations, but the degree of protection they provide varies widely. Although most state provisions are less protective than GINA, some are more protective. All entities that are subject to GINA must, at a minimum, comply with all applicable GINA requirements, and they may also need to comply with more protective state laws.

In conjunction with HIPAA, GINA generally prohibits health insurers or health plan administrators from requesting or requiring genetic information of an individual or the individual's family members, or using it for decisions regarding coverage, rates, or preexisting conditions. Employers are also prohibited from using genetic information for hiring, firing, or promotion decisions, and for any decisions regarding terms of employment.

The federal statute has attempted to more clearly define "genetic information" and does not include information about the sex or age of any individual (**Table 21-3**). A **genetic test** is defined as an analysis of human DNA, RNA, chromosomes, proteins, or

**Table 21-3  Definition of Genetic Information According to the Genetic Information Nondiscrimination Act of 2008**

An individual's genetic tests (including genetic tests done as part of a research study)

Genetic tests of the individual's family members (defined as dependents and up to and including fourth-degree relatives)

Genetic tests of any fetus of an individual or family member who is a pregnant woman, and genetic tests of any embryo legally held by an individual or family member utilizing assisted reproductive technology

The manifestation of a disease or disorder in family members (family history)

Any request for, or receipt of, genetic services or participation in clinical research that includes genetic services (genetic testing, counseling, or education) by an individual or family member

*Source:* Data from "Gina" The Genetic Information Nondiscrimination Act of 2008. Information for Researchers and Health Care Professionals. April 6, 2009. U.S. Department of Health and Human Services. Available at http://www.genome.gov/Pages/PolicyEthics/GeneticDiscrimination/GINAInfoDoc.pdf. Accessed January 18, 2010.

**Table 21-4   Areas That Are Not Protected by the Genetic Information Nondiscrimination Act of 2008**

Health coverage nondiscrimination protections do not extend to life insurance, disability insurance, and long-term care insurance.

The act does not mandate coverage for any particular test or treatment.

Employment provisions generally do not apply to employers with fewer than 15 employees.

For health coverage provided by a health insurer to individuals, the act does not prohibit the health insurer from determining eligibility or premium rates for an individual based on the manifestation of a disease or disorder in that individual.

For employment-based coverage provided by group health plans, the act permits the overall premium rate for an employer to be increased because of the manifestation of a disease or disorder of an individual enrolled in the plan, but the manifested disease or disorder of one individual cannot be used as genetic information about other group members to further increase the premium.

The act does not prohibit health insurers or health plan administrators from obtaining and using genetic test results in making health insurance payment determinations.

*Source:* Data from "Gina" The Genetic Information Nondiscrimination Act of 2008. Information for Researchers and Health Care Professionals. April 6, 2009. U.S. Department of Health and Human Services. Available at http://www.genome.gov/Pages/PolicyEthics/GeneticDiscrimination/GINAInfoDoc.pdf. Accessed January 18, 2010.

metabolites that detects genotypes, mutations, or chromosomal changes (Current Genetic Definitions in Minnesota Statutes and Federal Law, 2010). Routine laboratory tests that do not measure these genetic parameters (e.g., complete blood count, lipid tests, and liver function tests) are not protected under GINA. Specific information is also provided detailing what GINA will not do (**Table 21-4**).

## Conclusion

Almost all advances in scientific knowledge have brought with them ethical dilemmas. All healthcare providers need to be aware of the following principles of bioethics (adapted from Westman, 2006):

- Autonomy
  - Adults' right and ability to make their own decisions
  - Right to informed consent and confidentiality
  - Right not to know
- Beneficence
  - Act to improve the patient's welfare
- Nonmaleficence
  - Do no harm

- Justice
  - Fairness and equal access to care

While genetic research offers much promise for improving health, we are currently engaged in a transitional period between new discoveries and an understanding of how that knowledge will be applied. The main question is, How will we apply our new knowledge without violating the basic rights and privileges of individuals? It is likely that the Human Genome Project will be recorded in history as one of the greatest accomplishments of this century. The knowledge and research present no real danger in and of themselves. How their use is shaped and guided by policy, legislation, morals, and ethics, however, is critical.

It is imperative that genetic information be protected to prevent widespread discrimination against individuals and families by insurers, employers, and third-party payers. Because not all genetic tests have the same predictive value and because most genetic diseases have been determined to be multifactorial in origin, utilizing a genetic test to deny coverage and discriminate does not make sense scientifically. Moreover, as a matter of social justice, it is unfair to deny coverage based on a speculative system that we have just begun to understand.

As pointed out by Kahn, health insurance is not only a precious commodity for those who have coverage, but a limited resource shared by the community. The entire insurance industry is based on the prediction of illness, injury, disability, or death. If those consumers who are likely to make claims can be eliminated, then the insurance companies will become nothing more than businesses operating on the principle of charging higher premiums to provide less coverage to more consumers.

Even though there has been much excitement regarding the potential applications of the information gleaned from the human genome, it is imperative that we as a society proceed with extreme caution. For members of the healthcare industry, a top priority has to be protecting the confidentiality of genetic information for our patients and their families. As healthcare providers, we need to be vigorous advocates for our patients and protect them as much as possible from unwarranted discrimination by outside entities such as insurance companies, employers, and government agencies. Therefore, in addition to expecting their caregivers to possess excellent clinical and diagnostic skills, our patients will rely on providers more and more in the future to guide them through the potentially complex maze of genetic diseases and genetic testing.

To obtain more up-to-date information regarding ethical, legal, and social issues, the following Web sites are recommended:

- Genome.gov: http://www.genome.gov/10001618
- Genetics Home Reference: http://ghr.nlm.nih.gov/handbook/hgp/elsi
- Human Genome Project Information: http://www.ornl.gov/sci/techresources/ Human_Genome/research/elsi.shtml

## Chapter Summary

- Genetic information and testing will play an increasingly larger role in the screening, diagnosing, and treatment of disease.

- There is justifiable concern that sensitive genetic information might be used by insurance companies and employers to discriminate against certain individuals.

- As genetic testing for disease susceptibility becomes incorporated into clinical practice to a greater extent, primary care providers will increasingly initiate genetic counseling and referrals for testing.

- Genetic testing should not be performed until patients have received genetic counseling.

- The Genetic Information Nondiscrimination Act of 2008 provides a baseline level of protection against genetic discrimination for all Americans beyond those associated with the Health Insurance Portability and Accountability Act of 1996 and many state laws.

## Key Terms

**Genetic Information Nondiscrimination Act of 2008 (GINA):** federal legislation that provides a baseline level of protection against genetic discrimination for all Americans.

**Genetic test:** an analysis of human DNA, RNA, chromosomes, proteins, or metabolites that is intended to detect genotypes, mutations, or chromosomal changes.

## Chapter Review Questions

1. _____ is associated with many ethical, social, and legal concerns that need to be addressed during the counseling process.

2. Ideally, genetic testing begins with a _____ who has a diagnosis of the disease in question to determine if a responsible mutation can be found.

3. Potential benefits of genetic testing typically include _____, _____, and _____ that may reduce risk.

4. Patients need to fully understand that a positive genetic test result only represents a _____ and does not necessarily guarantee that they will get that disease.

5. _____ generally prohibits health insurers or health plan administrators from requesting or requiring genetic information of an individual or the individual's family members, or using it for decisions regarding coverage, rates, or preexisting conditions.

## Resources

Centre for Genetics Education, Fact Sheet 23. Some Ethical Issues in Genetics. http://www.genetics.com.au/pdf/factsheets/fs23.pdf.

Clayton EW. Ethical, Legal, and Social Implications of Genomic Medicine. *New England Journal of Medicine.* 349:562–569; 2003.

Collins FS, Green E, Guttmacher AE, Guyer MS. A Vision for the Future of Genomics Research. *Nature.* 422:835–847; 2003. http://www.genome.gov/11007524.

Current Genetic Definitions in Minnesota Statutes and Federal Law. Available at: http://www.ipad.state.mn.us/docs/geninfo22.pdf. Accessed January 27, 2010.

"GINA": The Genetic Information Nondiscrimination Act of 2008. Information for Researchers and Health Care Professionals. http://www.genome.gov/Pages/Poli cyEthics/GeneticDiscrimination/GINAInfoDoc.pdf.

Guidance on the Genetic Information Nondiscrimination Act: Implications for Investigators and Institutional Review Boards. Office for Human Research Protections, Department of Health and Human Services. http://www.hhs.gov/ohrp/humansubjects/guidance/gina.html.

Gunder LM. *Ethical Considerations in Medical Genetics* [Unpublished paper]. Fort Lauderdale, FL: Nova Southeastern University; 2006.

Kahn JP. Genetic testing: The Future Is Here. http://www.cnn.com/HEALTH/bio ethics/9808/genetics.part1/.

Kahn JP. Genetic Testing Aand Insurance. http://www.cnn.com/HEALTH/bioethics/9808/genetics.part2/template.html.

Westman JA. *Medical Genetics for the Modern Clinician.* Philadelphia: Lippincott Williams & Wilkins; 2006.

White MT, Callif-Daley F, Donnelly J. Genetic Testing for Disease Susceptibility: Social, Ethical and Legal Issues for Family Physicians. *American Family Physician.* 60:748, 750, 755, 757–758; 1999.

# Glossary

**Acquired hemophilia:** production of autoantibody that inactivates coagulation factors (VIII or IX) and results in the same clinical bleeding diathesis as occurs in inherited hemophilias.

**Acquired von Willebrand's disease:** a form of von Willebrand's disease that is not inherited but rather develops late in life. It is caused by the development of antibodies that attack and destroy a person's von Willebrand factor. This disease is commonly "acquired" in conjunction with another serious disease.

**Acute-phase reactant:** any substance that can be elevated in inflammatory processes.

**Adeno-associated virus:** any of a class of small, single-stranded DNA viruses that can insert their genetic material at a specific site on chromosome 19. Parvovirus is an example of this type of virus.

**Adenoma:** a benign epithelial neoplasm in which the tumor cells form glands or gland-like structures.

**Adenomatous:** relating to an adenoma, and to some types of glandular hyperplasia.

**Adenomatous polyposis coli (APC):** a tumor suppressor gene on chromosome 5. Mutations in this gene result in familial adenomatous polyposis.

**Adenovirus:** any of a class of viruses that contain double-stranded DNA and cause respiratory, intestinal, and eye infections in humans.

**Allele:** any one of a series of one, two, or more alternative forms of a gene that may occupy the same locus on a specific chromosome.

**Allelic variant:** an alteration in the normal sequence of a gene.

**Alpha-fetoprotein (AFP):** a protein product normally produced only in the fetal liver and used as a tumor marker in adults.

**Amniocentesis:** a prenatal test in which a small sample of the amniotic fluid surrounding the fetus is removed and examined.

**Amnion:** a membrane that forms a fluid-filled sac around the embryo.

**Amsterdam criteria:** research criteria for defining Lynch syndrome established by the International Collaborative Group meeting in Amsterdam.

**Anemia:** any condition in which the number of red blood cells per cubic millimeter ($mm^3$), the amount of hemoglobin in 100 mL of blood, and/or the volume of packed red blood cells per 100 mL of blood are less than normal.

**Aneuploidy:** a condition in which extra or fewer copies of particular genes or chromosomal regions are present compared with the wild type.

**Angina:** chest pain that is precipitated by exertion and relieved by rest; it is caused by inadequate oxygen delivery to the heart muscles.

**Anticipation:** the predictability of progressively earlier onset and increased severity of certain diseases in successive generations of affected persons.

**Aortic aneurysm:** an abnormal dilation of the aorta at the level of the ascending aorta or the sinuses of Valsalva (descending aorta).

**Aortic dissection:** a longitudinal tear between the layers of the aorta that may progress due to the high-pressure flow inside the aorta.

**Aplastic anemia:** a total bone marrow failure characterized by a decrease in all blood cells.

**Apoptosis:** programmed or gene-directed cell death.

**Arcus corneus:** a corneal disease caused by deposits of phospholipids and cholesterol in the corneal stroma and anterior sclera surrounding the iris of the eye.

**Atherosclerosis:** thickening and loss of elasticity of arterial walls, caused by lipid deposition and thickening of the intimal cell layers within arteries.

**Autoantibody:** a protein that attacks the body's own tissues.

**Autosomal dominant:** a pattern of inheritance in which an affected individual has one copy of a mutant gene and one normal gene on a pair of autosomal chromosomes. Individuals with autosomal dominant diseases have a 50:50 chance of passing the mutant gene—and, therefore, the disorder—on to each of their children.

**Autosomes:** all chromosomes other than the sex chromosomes.

**Azoospermia:** the absence of spermatozoa in the semen.

**Biliary cirrhosis:** cirrhosis due to biliary obstruction, which may be a primary intrahepatic disease or occur secondary to obstruction of extrahepatic bile ducts.

**Blast cells:** an immature precursor cell (e.g., erythroblast, lymphoblast, neuroblast).

**Blast crisis:** in a leukemic patient, a disease stage characterized by fever, fatigue, and clinically poor response to interventions.

**Blastocyst:** an early stage of embryo development, which can be recognized through the presence of an inner cell mass.

**Bleeding diathesis:** a group of distinct conditions in which a person's body cannot properly develop a clot, resulting in an increased tendency for bleeding.

**BRCA1:** a tumor suppressor gene on chromosome 17 that prevents cells with damaged DNA from dividing. Carriers of germline mutations in *BRCA1* are predisposed to develop both breast and ovarian cancer.

**BRCA2:** a tumor suppressor gene on chromosome 13. Carriers of germline mutations in *BRCA2* have an increased risk, similar to that of carriers of *BRCA1* mutations, of developing breast cancer and a moderately increased risk of ovarian cancer. *BRCA2* families also exhibit an increased incidence of male breast, pancreatic, prostate, laryngeal, and ocular cancers.

**Café-au-lait spot:** a flat spot on the skin that is the color of coffee with milk (café au lait) in persons with light skin. These spots are harmless by themselves, but in some cases they may be a sign of neurofibromatosis. The presence of six or more café-au-lait spots, each of which is 1.5 centimeters or more in diameter, is diagnostic for neurofibromatosis.

**Cardiomyopathy:** a disease of the myocardium (heart muscle) that has variable etiologies and clinical presentations; any condition in which the myocardium is dysfunctional.

**Carrier:** a person (usually female) who can pass an altered gene to her children, but generally does not express the disease herself; a term used to describe heterozygotes in recessive disorders who do not express disease characteristics themselves but can pass the mutation on to their offspring.

**Cephalohematoma:** a collection of blood under the skull due to an effusion of blood, usually as a result of trauma.

**CFTR gene:** a gene that codes for a protein involved in chloride and water transport across membranes. In patients with cystic fibrosis, a mutation in this gene disrupts chloride and water transport across membranes. The end result is production of thick and sticky mucus that obstructs the airways in the lungs and the ducts in the pancreas.

**Cholesterol:** the principal sterol found in all higher animals. It is distributed in body tissues, especially the brain and spinal cord, and in animal fats and oils.

**Chorea:** from the Greek word for "dance"; the incessant, quick, jerky, involuntary movements that are characteristic of Huntington's disease.

**Chorionic villus sampling (CVS):** a prenatal test that involves taking a tiny tissue sample from outside the sac where the fetus develops. It is performed between 10 and 12 weeks after a now-pregnant woman's last menstrual period.

**Chromosomal aberration:** alteration in the number or physical structure of chromosomes.

**Chromosome:** a DNA molecule that contains genes in linear order to which numerous proteins are bound.

**Chromosome painting:** use of differentially labeled, chromosome-specific DNA strands for hybridization with chromosomes to label each chromosome with a different color.

**Chronic myelogenous leukemia (CML):** a myeloproliferative disorder characterized by increased proliferation of the granulocytic cell line without the loss of their capacity to differentiate.

**Cirrhosis:** a degenerative disease of the liver characterized by formation of fibrous tissue and scarring, resulting in the inhibition of normal cellular function.

**Clotting factor:** any of several proteins that are involved in the blood coagulation process.

**Coagulation:** the chemical reaction mediated by coagulation factor proteins that results in a stable fibrin clot.

**Codon:** a sequence of three adjacent nucleotides in an mRNA molecule, specifying either an amino acid or a stop signal in protein synthesis.

**Colectomy:** surgical excision of part or all of the colon.

**Computed tomography (CT) scan:** an imaging procedure that makes a series of detailed pictures of areas inside the body, taken from different angles by using a computer linked to an x-ray machine.

**Consanguinity:** degree of relationship between persons who descend from a common ancestor.

**Consanguineous:** mating between related individuals.

**Cor pulmonale:** failure of the right ventricle of the heart, secondary to enlargement and increased pressure caused by disease of the lungs or pulmonary blood vessels.

**Covariates:** the interplay of environmental factors with genetic predisposition.

**Cowden syndrome:** a cancer syndrome inherited in an autosomal dominant pattern that manifests as neoplasms of the skin, thyroid, mucosa, gastrointestinal tract, bones, eyes, and genitourinary tract. The most common mutation is found in the *PTEN* gene.

**Crowe sign:** axillary and inguinal freckling, often associated with type 1 neurofibromatosis.

**Cystic fibrosis:** a congenital metabolic disorder, inherited as an autosomal recessive trait, in which secretions of exocrine glands are abnormal. Excessively viscid mucus causes obstruction of passageways (including pancreatic and bile ducts, intestines, and bronchi), and the sodium and chloride content of sweat are increased throughout the patient's life

**Cystic fibrosis–related diabetes mellitus:** insulin deficiency and insulin resistance caused by complications from cystic fibrosis.

**De novo mutations:** mutations that are not inherited, but rather appear first in the affected individual.

**Degenerate:** a feature of the genetic code in which an amino acid corresponds to more than one codon.

**Deletion:** absence of a segment of DNA; it may be as small as a single base or large enough to encompass one or more entire genes. Any spontaneous elimination of part of the normal genetic complement, whether cytogenetically visible (chromosomal deletion) or found by molecular techniques.

**Deoxyribonucleic acid (DNA):** a macromolecule usually composed of two polynucleotide chains in a double helix that is the carrier of genetic information in all cells.

**Desmopressin acetate:** a synthetic hormone that increases factor VIII levels.

**Disseminated intravascular coagulation:** a condition of altered coagulation that results in consumption of clotting factors and platelets and yields a clinical presentation characterized by both excessive clotting and excessive bleeding.

**Diverticula:** a pouch or sac opening from a tubular or saccular organ such as the intestines or the bladder.

**Diverticulitis:** inflammation of a diverticulum, especially of the small pockets in the wall of the colon, which fill with stagnant fecal material and become inflamed. Rarely, these sacs may cause obstruction, perforation, or bleeding.

**Dominant:** refers to an allele whose presence in a heterozygous genotype results in a phenotype characteristic of the allele.

**Dominant negative mutation:** a mutated allele that disrupts the function of a normal allele in the same cell.

**Down syndrome:** a chromosomal dysgenesis syndrome consisting of a variable constellation of abnormalities caused by triplication or translocation of chromosome 21. Affected individuals have some degree of mental retardation, characteristic facial features, and, often, heart defects and other health problems.

**Dyskinesia:** difficulty in performing voluntary movements.

**Ectoderm:** the outer layer of cells in the embryo, after establishment of the three primary germ layers (ectoderm, mesoderm, endoderm); the germ layer that comes in contact with the amniotic cavity.

**Embryo:** the developing human within the first two months after conception.

**End-stage renal disease (ESRD):** the complete or almost complete failure of the kidneys to function. The dysfunctional kidneys can no longer remove wastes, concentrate urine, and regulate electrolytes.

**Endoderm:** the innermost of the three primary germ layers of the embryo (ectoderm, mesoderm, endoderm). The epithelial lining of the primitive gut tract and the epithelial component of the glands and other structures (e.g., lower respiratory system) that develop as outgrowths from the gut tube are derived from the endoderm.

**Ethnic variation of allelic frequency:** a situation which frequency of mutated alleles is higher among certain ethnic groups than in others.

**Fabry disease:** an inherited lipid storage disease that results from a deficiency in the enzyme alpha-galactosidase found on the X chromosome. This defect leads to the accumulation of glycospingolipids in the plasma and lysosomes of vascular endothelial and smooth muscle cells.

**Factor assay:** a specialized lab test used to determine the level of circulating factor VIII or IX.

**Factor deficiency:** any of several rare disorders characterized by the complete absence or an abnormally low level of clotting factor in the blood.

**Factor inhibitors:** antibodies that develop in patients in response to factor replacement therapy.

**Factor replacement therapy:** replacement of a deficient clotting factor from another source (either human derived or recombinant) in an effort to stop or prevent abnormal bleeding.

**Familial adenomatous polyposis (FAP):** an inherited colorectal cancer syndrome that leads to hundreds—sometimes even thousands—of polyps in the colon and rectum at a young age.

**Fetal alcohol effect:** the development of relatively mild degrees of mental deficiency and emotional disorders in children whose mothers use alcohol during their pregnancy; this condition is more common than the full fetal alcohol syndrome scenario.

**Fifth disease:** a disease caused by infection with human parvovirus B19, which infects only humans. It manifests as a mild rash illness that occurs most commonly in children. The ill child typically has a "slapped-cheek" rash on the face and a lacy red rash on the trunk and limbs.

**First-degree relative:** any relative who is one meiosis away from a particular individual in a family (i.e., parent, sibling, offspring).

**Fluorescence in situ hybridization (FISH):** a analytic technique in which a nucleic acid labeled with a fluorescent dye is hybridized to suitably prepared cells or histological sections; it is then used to look for specific transcription or localization of genes to specific chromosomes.

**Founder effect:** accumulation of random genetic changes in an isolated population as a result of its proliferation from only a few parent colonizers.

**Frameshift mutation:** an insertion or deletion involving a number of base pairs that is not a multiple of three and consequently disrupts the triplet reading frame, usually leading to the creation of a premature termination (stop) codon and resulting in a truncated protein product.

**Gain-of-function mutation:** a genetic change that increases the activity of a gene protein or increases the production of the protein.

**Gene:** a region of DNA containing genetic information, which is usually transcribed into an RNA molecule that is processed and either functions directly or is translated into a polypeptide chain; the hereditary unit.

**Genetic heterogeneity:** the production of the same or similar phenotypes by different genetic mechanisms; the character of a phenotype produced by mutation at more than one gene or by more than one genetic mechanism.

**Genetic Information Nondiscrimination Act of 2008 (GINA):** federal legislation that provides a baseline level of protection against genetic discrimination for all Americans.

**Genetic test:** an analysis of human DNA, RNA, chromosomes, proteins, or metabolites that is intended to detect genotypes, mutations, or chromosomal changes.

**Genocopy:** a genotype that determines a phenotype which closely resembles the phenotype determined by a different genotype.

**Genomics:** systematic study of an organism's genome using large-scale DNA sequencing, gene-expression analysis, or computational methods.

**Germinal mutation:** a mutation that takes place in a reproductive cell.

**Germline mutation:** a change in a gene in the body's reproductive cell (egg or sperm) that becomes incorporated into the DNA of every cell in the body of the offspring.

**Glioma:** any neoplasm derived from one of the various types of cells that form the interstitial tissue of the brain, spinal cord, pineal gland, posterior pituitary gland, and retina.

**Granulocyte:** a mature granular leukocyte, including any of the neutrophilic, acidophilic, and basophilic types of polymorphonuclear leukocytes (i.e., neutrophils, eosinophils, and basophils).

**Hamartoma:** a focal malformation that resembles a neoplasm, grossly and even microscopically, but results from faulty development in an organ.

**Head and neck squamous cell carcinoma:** cancer originating from the mucosal lining (epithelium) of the head and neck.

**Hemarthroses:** bleeding into joints.

**Hematoma:** bleeding into soft tissue, such as muscle or visceral organs.

**Hemizygous:** describes an individual who has only one member of a chromosome pair or chromosome segment rather than the usual two; refers in particular to X-linked genes in males who under usual circumstances have only one X chromosome.

**Hemoglobin C disease:** a type of hemoglobin-related disease characterized by episodes of abdominal and joint pain, an enlarged spleen, and mild jaundice, but no severe crises. This disease occurs mostly in African Americans, who may show few symptoms of its presence.

**Hemoglobin SC disease:** a type of hemoglobin-related disease that occurs in people who have one copy of the gene for sickle cell disease and one copy of the gene for hemoglobin C disease.

**Hemophilia:** a bleeding disorder in which a specific clotting factor protein—namely, factor VIII or IX—is missing or does not function normally.

**Hemophilia A:** a deficiency or absence of factor VIII; also been called "classic" hemophilia. It is the most common severe bleeding disorder.

**Hemophilia B:** a deficiency or absence of factor IX; also called "Christmas disease" after the first family that was identified with the condition.

**Hemophilia B Leyden:** a rare variant of hemophilia B inherited in an X-linked pattern.

**Hemophilia C:** a deficiency or absence of factor XI; more commonly known as plasma thromboplastin antecedent deficiency.

**Hemophilia treatment centers:** a group of federally funded hospitals that specialize in treating patients with coagulation disorders.

**Hemostasis:** the process by which the body stops bleeding.

**Hepatic ultrasound:** an imaging study of the liver used to detect the presence of tissue changes such as tumors, abscesses, and cysts.

**Hepatitis:** inflammation of the liver causing impaired function as a result of toxins (e.g., alcohol, iron, drugs), autoimmune disorders, or infectious agents (viruses).

**Hepatoma:** the most common type of non-metastatic liver cancer; also known as primary hepatocellular carcinoma.

**Hepatomegaly:** enlargement of the liver.

**Hepatotoxic:** relating to an agent that damages the liver.

**Hereditary hemochromatosis:** an autosomal recessive disorder caused by a single mutation in the HFE gene, which causes increased intestinal absorption of iron and results in increased iron storage in body tissues

**Hereditary nonpolyposis colorectal cancer (HNPCC):** an inherited colorectal cancer syndrome in which only a small number of polyps are present or not present at all. Also known as Lynch syndrome.

**Herpes simplex virus:** any of a class of double-stranded DNA viruses that infect a particular cell type, specifically the neurons.

**Heterozygote advantage:** a mutated allele at the same locus as a normal allele that confers the advantage of protection against a disease and increases survival.

**Heterozygous:** carrying dissimilar alleles of one or more genes; not homozygous.

**Homozygous:** having the same allele of a gene in homologous chromosomes.

**Human leukocyte antigen (HLA):** system designation for the gene products of at least four linked loci (A, B, C, and D) and a number of subloci on the sixth human chromosome that have been shown to have a strong influence on human allotransplantation, transfusions in refractory patients, and certain disease associations. More than 50 alleles are recognized, most of which are found at loci HLA-A and HLA-B; they are passed on through autosomal dominant inheritance.

**Huntingtin:** the product of the Huntington's disease gene on chromosome 4.

**Hydrocephalus:** a condition marked by an excessive accumulation of cerebrospinal fluid, resulting in dilation of the cerebral ventricles and raised intracranial pressure; it may also result in enlargement of the cranium and atrophy of the brain.

**Hypertrichosis:** growth of hair in excess of the normal.

**Inborn errors of metabolism:** a genetically determined biochemical disorder, usually in the form of an enzyme defect that produces a metabolic block.

**Inner cell mass (ICM):** the cells at the embryonic pole of the blastocyst, which are concerned with formation of the body of the embryo.

**Insertion:** a chromosome abnormality in which material from one chromosome is inserted into another nonhomologous chromosome; a mutation in which a segment of DNA is inserted into a gene or other segment of DNA, potentially disrupting the coding sequence.

**International Normalized Ratio (INR):** a system established by the World Health Organization and the International Committee on Thrombosis and Hemostasis for reporting the results of blood coagulation (clotting) tests. All results are standardized using the international sensitivity index for the particular thromboplastin reagent and instrument combination used to perform the test. No matter which laboratory checks the prothrombin time, the result should be the same even if different thromboplastins and instruments are used.

**Inversion:** a structural aberration in a chromosome in which the order of several genes is reversed from the normal order.

**Iris flocculi:** an ocular abnormality found in persons with familial thoracic aortic aneurysms and dissections that is highly associated with *ACTA2* mutations.

**Karyotype:** the chromosome complement of a cell or organism; often represented by an arrangement of metaphase chromosomes according to their lengths and the positions of their centromeres.

**Kindred:** an aggregate of genetically related persons.

**Klinefelter syndrome:** a disorder that occurs when an ovum with an extra X chromosome is fertilized by a sperm with a Y chromosome. This results in an XXY genotype male who is sterile.

**Left ventricular hypertrophy (LVH):** enlargement of the muscle tissue in the wall of the left ventricle, often involving the intra-ventricular septum.

**Lentivirus:** a type of complex retrovirus that can enter nondividing cells through pores in the nuclear membrane. Human immunodeficiency virus is an example.

**Li-Fraumeni syndrome:** is a rare syndrome associated with a germline mutation on chromosome 17. It is characterized by premenopausal breast cancer in combination with childhood sarcoma, brain tumors, leukemia, and adrenocortical carcinoma. Tumors in families who carry the Li-Fraumeni syndrome mutation tend to occur in childhood and early adulthood and often present as multiple primary tumors in the same individual. The average age of onset of breast cancer is 34.6 years in families with this mutation.

**Liposome:** an artificial lipid sphere with an aqueous core.

**Lisch nodule:** iris hamartomas, typically seen in type 1 neurofibromatosis.

**Livedo reticularis:** a purplish skin discoloration in a lacy pattern caused by constriction of deep dermal capillaries.

**Locus:** the site or position of a particular gene on a chromosome.

**Loss-of-function mutation:** a genetic change that reduces the activity of a gene protein or decreases the production of the protein; insertion of the normal gene corrects this defect.

**Low-density lipoprotein:** the type of lipoprotein responsible for transport of cholesterol to extrahepatic tissues.

**Lymph node mapping:** a procedure in which a radioactive substance or blue dye is injected near the tumor, then flows through lymph ducts to the first lymph node or nodes where cancer cells are likely to have spread. Lymph nodes that are marked with the dye are then surgically removed and examined microscopically by a pathologist for evidence of cancer cells.

**Magnetic resonance imaging (MRI):** a procedure that uses a magnet, radio waves, and a computer to make a series of detailed images of areas inside the body.

**Marfan syndrome:** a connective tissue, multisystemic disorder characterized by skeletal changes (arachnodactyly, long limbs, joint laxity), cardiovascular defects (aortic aneurysm that may dissect, mitral valve prolapse), and ectopia lentis. It is passed on through autosomal dominant inheritance of a mutation in the fibrillin-1 gene on chromosome 15.

**Meconium ileus:** obstruction of the intestines due to retention of a dark green waste product (meconium) that is normally passed shortly after a child's birth.

**Melanomagenesis:** the formation of melanoma.

**Mendelian genetics:** the mechanism of inheritance in which the statistical relations between the distribution of traits in successive generations result from three factors: (1) particulate hereditary determinants (genes), (2) random union of gametes, and (3) segregation of unchanged hereditary determinants in the reproductive cells.

**Menorrhagia:** excessive bleeding during the time of menses, in terms of either duration or volume, or both.

**Merlin:** a tumor suppressor gene encoded on chromosome 22 (*NF2* gene). Mutation of this gene disrupts tumor suppressor activity and leads to the formation of schwannomas associated with type 2 neurofibromatosis.z

**Mesoderm:** the middle of the three primary germ layers of the embryo (the others being ectoderm and endoderm). The mesoderm is the origin of connective tissues, myoblasts, blood, the cardiovascular and lymphatic systems, most of the urogenital system, and the lining of the pericardial, pleural, and peritoneal cavities.

**Messenger ribonucleic acid (mRNA):** an RNA molecule that is transcribed from a DNA sequence and translated into the amino acid sequence of a polypeptide.

**Microcephaly:** abnormal smallness of the head; a term applied to a skull with a capacity of less than 1350 mL. Microcephaly is usually associated with mental retardation.

**Microfibrils:** structural molecules found in load-bearing tissues.

**Microsatellite instability:** a change that occurs in the DNA of certain cells (e.g., tumor cells) in which the number of repeats of microsatellites (short, repeated sequences of DNA) is different than the number of repeats that appeared in the DNA when it was inherited. The cause of microsatellite instability may be a defect in the ability to repair mistakes made when DNA is copied in the cell.

**Mild hemophilia:** a categorical term used to describe someone with a factor VIII or IX level ranging between 5% and 25% of normal blood levels.

**Missense mutation:** a mutation in which a base change or substitution results in a codon that causes insertion of a different amino acid into the growing polypeptide chain, giving rise to an altered protein.

**Mitochondrial chromosome:** a small circular chromosome found in each mitochondrion that encodes tRNA, rRNA, and proteins that are involved in oxidative phosphorylation and ATP generation.

**Moderate hemophilia:** a categorical term used to describe someone with a factor VIII or IX level ranging between 1% and 5% of normal blood levels.

**Monogenic:** of, relating to, or controlled by a single gene, especially by either of an allelic pair.

**Monosomy:** a condition in an otherwise diploid organism in which one member of a pair of chromosomes is missing.

**Morning after pill:** a form of emergency birth control used to prevent a woman from becoming pregnant after she has engaged in unprotected vaginal intercourse.

**Morula:** the earliest stage of embryo after cell division, consisting of a ball of identical cells.

**Mutation:** heritable alteration in a gene or chromosome; also, the process by which such an alteration happens.

**Myelodysplastic syndrome:** the underproduction of a single type of blood cell produced in the bone marrow.

**Myelofibrosis:** fibrosis of the bone marrow associated with myeloid metaplasia of the spleen and other organs.

**Myocardial infarction:** death of the heart muscle, caused by occlusion of the coronary vessels.

**Myocardium:** the heart muscle cells responsible for contractility of the heart.

**Neoplastic:** related to the pathologic process that results in the formation and growth of a neoplasm or abnormal tissue that may be either benign or malignant.

**Nephrotoxic:** relating to an agent that damages renal cells.

**Neurofibroma:** a benign, encapsulated tumor resulting from proliferation of Schwann cells that are of ectodermal (neural crest) origin and that form a continuous envelope around each nerve fiber of peripheral nerves.

**Neurofibromin:** a tumor suppressor gene encoded on chromosome 17 (*NF1* gene). Loss of tumor suppression due to a mutation in this gene leads to the formation of neurofibromas associated with type 1 neurofibromatosis.

**Nondisjunction:** failure of chromosomes to separate (disjoin) and move to opposite poles of the division spindle; the result is loss or gain of a chromosome.

**Nonsense mutation:** a single base-pair substitution that prematurely codes for a stop in amino acid translation (stop codon).

**Novel property mutation:** a mutation that confers a new property on the protein product.

**Oligonucleotide:** a DNA sequence consisting of a small number of nucleotide bases.

**Oncogene:** any of a family of genes that under normal circumstances code for proteins involved in cell growth or regulation (e.g., protein kinases), but that may foster malignant processes if mutated or activated by contact with retroviruses.

**Organogenesis:** formation of organs during development.

**Packaging cells:** cells in which replication-deficient viruses are placed so that the replication machinery of the packaging cell can produce viral copies.

**Paracrines:** a group of chemical messengers that communicate with neighboring cells by simple diffusion.

**Parturition:** the process of birth.

**Pedigree analysis:** a diagram representing the familial relationships among relatives.

**Penetrance:** the proportion of organisms having a particular genotype that actually express the corresponding phenotype. If the phenotype is always expressed, penetrance is complete; otherwise, it is incomplete.

**Peutz-Jeghers syndrome:** a disorder with known association to polyposis and adrenocarcinoma that manifests as dark-freckling around the mouth, eyes, and extremities, as well as increased incidence of intestinal polyps. There is also a five- to tenfold increased risk of testicular and ovarian neoplasia.

**Pharmacogenetics:** the study of the interrelation of hereditary constitution and response to drugs.

**Pharmacogenomics:** the combination of pharmacology and genomics in an effort to develop effective and safe medications in a ways that compensates for genetic differences in patients that cause varied responses to a single therapeutic regimen.

**Phenylalanine hydroxylase (PAH):** the enzyme that converts phenylalanine to tyrosine and that is defective in phenylketonuria.

**Phenylketonuria (PKU):** a hereditary human condition resulting from inability to convert phenylalanine into tyrosine. It causes severe mental retardation unless treated in infancy and childhood by a low-phenylalanine diet.

**Philadelphia chromosome:** an abnormal chromosome formed by a rearrangement of chromosomes 9 and 22 that is associated with chronic myelogenous leukemia.

**Phocomelia:** defective development of arms or legs, or both, so that the hands and feet are attached close to the body, resembling the flippers of a seal.

**Phototype:** a classification system based on a person's sensitivity to sunlight as measured by the ability to tan.

**Placenta:** a structure consisting of maternal and fetal tissues that allows for exchange of gases, nutrients, and wastes between the mother's circulatory system and the circulatory system of the fetus.

**Point mutation:** the alteration of a single nucleotide to a different nucleotide.

**Polycythemia vera:** a chronic form of polycythemia of unknown cause characterized by bone marrow hyperplasia, an increase in both blood volume and the number of red cells, redness or cyanosis of the skin, and splenomegaly.

**Polygenic:** genetic disorder resulting from the combined action of alleles of more than one gene.

**Polymerase chain reaction (PCR):** repeated cycles of DNA denaturation, renaturation with primer oligonucleotide sequences, and replication, resulting in exponential growth in the number of copies of the DNA sequence located between the primers.

**Polymorphisms:** natural variations in a gene, DNA sequence, or chromosome that have no adverse effects on the individual and occur with fairly high frequency in the general population.

**Polyp:** a usually nonmalignant growth or tumor protruding from the mucous lining of an organ such as the nose, bladder, or intestine, often causing obstruction.

**Polysomy:** condition of a diploid cell or organism that has three or more copies of a particular chromosome.

**Porencephaly:** the occurrence of cavities in the brain substance, communicating usually with the lateral ventricles.

**Portal hypertension:** elevation of pressure in the hepatic portal circulation due to cirrhosis or other fibrotic change in liver tissue. When pressure exceeds 10 mm Hg, a collateral circulation may develop to maintain venous return from structures drained by the portal vein; engorgement of collateral veins can lead to esophageal varices and, less often, caput medusae.

**Positron emission tomography (PET) scan:** an imaging procedure used to locate malignant tumor cells in the body by identifying areas of tissue with greatest glucose utilization.

**Proband:** an affected person as identified in a family pedigree.

**Probe:** a labeled DNA or RNA molecule used in DNA-RNA or DNA-DNA hybridization assays.

**Proctocolectomy:** a surgical procedure involving the excision of the colon and rectum and the formation of an ileoanal reservoir or pouch.

**Prodrug:** a class of drugs in which the pharmacologic action results from conversion by metabolic processes within the body.

**Prothrombin time:** a clotting test done to test the integrity of part of the clotting scheme, which is commonly used as a method of monitoring the accuracy of blood thinning treatment (anticoagulation) with warfarin. The test measures the time needed for clot formation after thromboplastin (plus calcium) has been added to plasma.

**Proto-oncogene:** a gene in the normal human genome that appears to have a role in normal cellular physiology and is involved in regulation of normal cell growth or proliferation; as a result of somatic mutations, these genes may become oncogenic.

**Recessive:** refers to an allele, or the corresponding phenotypic trait, that is expressed only in homozygotes.

**Recurrent melanoma:** cancer that has returned after it has been treated to either the original site or in other areas of the body.

**Renal cell carcinoma:** a type of kidney cancer in which the cancerous cells are found in the lining of very small tubes (tubules) in the kidney.

**Ribosomal RNA (rRNA):** a type of RNA molecule that is a component of the ribosomal subunits.

**Ribozymes:** RNA molecules with enzyme activity that can cleave messenger RNA.

**Sarcomere:** the simplest unit of muscle tissue that allows the muscle to contract.

**Satellite moles:** new moles that grow in a pattern around existing moles.

**Schwannoma:** a benign, encapsulated neoplasm in which the fundamental component is structurally identical to a syncytium of Schwann cells. The neoplasm may originate from a peripheral or sympathetic nerve, or from various cranial nerves, particularly the eighth nerve.

**Sentinel node:** the first lymph node to receive lymphatic drainage from a tumor.

**Serum ferritin levels:** a measure of the amount of iron bound to transferrin.

**Serum iron levels:** a measure of the amount of unbound iron that has been transported to the blood.

**Severe combined immune deficiency:** any of a group of rare, sometimes fatal, congenital disorders characterized by little or no immune response.

**Severe hemophilia:** a categorical term used to describe someone with a factor VIII or IX level that is less than 1% of normal blood levels.

**Sex chromosome:** a chromosome, such as the human X or Y, that plays a role in the determination of sex.

**Sex-influenced phenotype:** a phenotype expressed in both male and females but with different frequencies in the two sexes.

**Sibling (sib):** a brother or sister, each having the same parents.

**Sickle cell trait:** the heterozygous state of the gene for hemoglobin S in sickle cell anemia.

**Somatic mutation:** a mutation arising in a somatic cell.

**Spontaneous bleeding:** heavy bleeding without history of trauma.

**Steatorrhea:** excretion of excess fat in the feces.

**Synergistic hepatotoxic effects:** toxic effects that work together such that the total toxic effect is greater than the sum of the two (or more) single effects.

**Target cell:** an erythrocyte with a dark center surrounded by a light band that is encircled by a darker ring; thus it resembles a shooting target.

**Thalassemia:** any of a group of inherited disorders of hemoglobin metabolism in which there is impaired synthesis of one or more of the polypeptide chains of globin.

**Therapeutic phlebotomy:** removal of a portion of the blood volume to alleviate symptoms.

**Thoracic aortic aneurysm:** widening or bulging of the upper portion of the aorta that may occur in the descending thoracic aorta, the ascending aorta, or the aortic arch.

**Thrombocytopenia:** a condition in which an abnormally small number of platelets appear in the circulating blood.

**Thrombocythemia:** a primary form of thrombocytopenia, in contrast to secondary forms that are associated with metastatic neoplasms, tuberculosis, and leukemia involving the bone marrow, or occurring as the result of direct suppression of bone marrow by the use of chemical agents.

**Total iron-binding capacity (TIBC):** a measure of all proteins available to bind iron and an indirect measure of transferrin levels.

**Transcription:** the process by which the information contained in a template strand of DNA is copied into a single-stranded RNA molecule of complementary base sequence.

**Transduction:** transfer of genetic material (and its phenotypic expression) from one cell to another by viral infection.

**Transfer ribonucleic acids (tRNA):** a small RNA molecule that translates a codon into an amino acid in protein synthesis; it has a three-base sequence, called the anticodon, complementary to a specific codon in mRNA, and a site to which a specific amino acid is bound.

**Transferrin:** the globulin protein that transports iron to the bone marrow.

**Transferrin saturation levels:** the portion of transferrin bound to iron. This value is found by dividing the serum iron by the total iron binding capacity.

**Translation:** the process by which the amino acid sequence of a polypeptide is synthesized on a ribosome according to the nucleotide sequence of an mRNA molecule.

**Translocation:** a mutation results from an exchange of parts of two chromosomes.

**Triplet repeat expansion:** a condition in which the number of repeating triplet units in a gene is so great that it interferes with gene expression and causes more severe disease.

**Trisomy:** a disorder in which a normally diploid organism has an extra copy of one of the chromosomes.

**Trophoblast:** the cell layer covering the blastocyst that erodes the uterine mucosa and through which the embryo receives nourishment from the mother. The cells do not enter into the formation of the embryo itself, but rather contribute to the formation of the placenta.

**Truncated protein:** a protein that does not achieve its full length or its proper form, and thus is missing some of the amino acid residues that are present in a normal protein. A truncated protein generally cannot perform the function for which it was intended because its structure is incapable of doing so.

**Tumor suppressor gene:** a gene whose function is to suppress cellular proliferation; a gene that encodes a protein involved in controlling cellular growth. Loss of a tumor suppressor gene through chromosomal aberration leads to heightened susceptibility to neoplasia.

**Tumorigenesis:** production of a new growth or growths.

**Turner syndrome:** a monosomy syndrome that results when an ovum lacking the X chromosome is fertilized by a sperm that contains an X chromosome. It may also occur when a genetically normal ovum is fertilized by a sperm lacking an X or Y chromosome. The result is an offspring with 22 pairs of autosomes and a single, unmatched X chromosome.

**Variable expressivity:** variation in disease symptoms among persons with the same mutation.

**Varices:** an enlarged and tortuous vein, artery, or lymphatic vessel.

**Vector:** the vehicle used to carry a DNA insert (e.g., a virus).

**Von Willebrand's disease:** a bleeding disorder in which von Willebrand factor, a blood protein, is either missing or does not function properly. It is the most common congenital bleeding disorder in the United States.

**Wide local excision:** a surgical procedure to remove some of the normal tissue surrounding the area where melanoma was found to check for cancer cells not visible on gross examination.

**Wolff-Parkinson-White syndrome:** an electrocardiographic pattern sometimes associated with paroxysmal tachycardia; it consists of a short P-R interval (usually 0.1 second or less; occasionally normal) together with a prolonged QRS complex with a slurred initial component (delta wave).

**X-linked recessive:** recessive inheritance pattern of alleles at loci on the X chromosome that do not undergo crossing over during male meiosis.

**Xanthomas:** a cutaneous manifestation of lipid accumulation in the large foam cells that presents clinically as small eruptions with distinct morphologies along tendons such as the Achilles tendon.

**Xanthelasmata:** sharply demarcated yellowish collections of cholesterol in foam cells observed underneath the skin and especially on the eyelids.

**Yolk sac:** the sac of extraembryonic membrane that is located ventral to the embryonic disk and, after formation of the gut tube, is connected to the midgut; by the second month of development, this connection has become the narrow yolk stalk. The yolk sac is the first hematopoietic organ of the embryo.

**Zygote:** fertilized ovum before cleavage begins.

# Index

NOTE: Page numbers with italicized *f* or *t* indicate figures or tables respectively.